LETHAL
SECRETS

LETHAL SECRETS

The Shocking Consequences
and Unsolved Problems of
Artificial Insemination

ANNETTE BARAN
and REUBEN PANNOR

WARNER BOOKS

A Warner Communications Company

AN AMISTAD BOOK

Warner Books, Inc., 666 Fifth Avenue, New York, NY 10103

W A Warner Communications Company

Printed in the United States of America
First printing April 1989
10 9 8 7 6 5 4 3 2 1

Library of Congress Cataloging-in-Publication Data

Baran, Annette.
  Lethal secrets : the shocking consequences and unsolved problems of
  artificial insemination / Annette Baran & Reuben Pannor.
      p. 208.
    Bibliography: p.
    Includes index.
    1. Artificial insemination, Human.   I. Pannor, Reuben.
  II. Title.
  RG134.B35   1989
  613.9'4—dc19   88-23670
  ISBN 0-446-71003-2   CIP

Designed by Giorgetta Bell McRee

*This book is dedicated to our families
and colleagues who have been forbearing
and supportive of our efforts to open doors
and eliminate secrecy in human relationships.*

CONTENTS

ACKNOWLEDGMENTS

This book is about a subject that remains largely secret. The people of the world of donor insemination have spent their lives with sealed lips and fears of disclosure. For them, therefore, to volunteer to participate in our study was courageous.

We are indebted to all of the individuals who shared their feelings with us. The married couples, donor fathers, donor offspring, lesbian couples, and single mothers who told us their stories made it possible for us to write this book. It was, for most of them, a first opportunity to talk about their experiences openly.

In our study we found ourselves in the position of being teacher, student, observer, researcher, analyst, and friend. We started our investigation with few strong convictions. We completed this book with an enormous sense of dedication to the need for fundamental change in the practice of donor insemination. Our contact and connection with all of the volunteers helped to develop our belief system. We hope that they gained as much from the experience as we did.

We also wish to thank all of the professionals and paraprofessionals who interviewed participants whom we could not reach. They were important to the scope of the study.

There are many reasons why people offer to participate in research studies. We know that an important reason stated over and over again by members of the donor insemination family, in our interviews, was the hope that the future for others in their situation would be different from the past. They hoped that they could help eliminate the painful and destructive secrecy surrounding their world.

We share that hope.

FOREWORD

The authors have provided a major breakthrough on a subject that has heretofore received scant attention from the scientific community. This despite the fact that the first documented report of insemination by a donor in the United States appeared in 1890. Subsequently, tens of thousands of anonymous and unknowing individuals have owed their lives to this secret procedure.

It has been assumed that individuals conceived through donor insemination should never be told of the true nature of their conception. At the same time, insemination donors were assured of their privacy and told that their identity would never be revealed. This practice of intentional deception has placed a strain on the parents. The burden of maintaining such a "family secret" has created many dysfunctional families and not infrequently led to divorce.

This monumental work has introduced a well-thought-out new nomenclature available for use by professionals and lay individuals alike in dealing with the practice of human insemination. A terminology is often the first step in clarifying a scientific venture. There is no doubt that such a direction is vital in developing a more objective insight into this very popular infertility-corrective procedure.

This work allows its readers to take a first peek at a hundred-year-old medical practice. Furthermore, questions are continuously raised that branch out into many nonmedical territories: psychological, sociological, ethical, religious, and legal. The reader is left to speculate on many of these issues because there are no hard answers to most of them. The provocative quality of this undertaking makes the book that much more intriguing.

We are now well entrenched in the era of alternative conception procedures. Donor insemination is the parent procedure, and work in this area will serve as a model in approaching other methods from a more highly rational and scientific standpoint. Such a focus is vital to the entire field of infertility medical psychology.

It will be essential that all of the issues raised herein receive careful consideration through further research and continuous evaluation and reevaluation. Follow-up studies are necessary to provide an insight into the long-term effects of donor insemination and to enable physicians and mental-health specialists to better screen and prepare their patients for the procedure.

The reader is about to embark upon a true literary adventure: entering uncharted waters and exploring their channels in company with all of the vigor and excitement of the social scientist.

ARTHUR D. SOROSKY, M.D.
Encino, California
July 22, 1988

LETHAL SECRETS

"Before I built a wall I'd ask to know
What I was walling in or walling out,
And to whom I was like to give offense.
Something there is
   that doesn't love a wall,
That wants it down."

From *Mending Wall*
by ROBERT FROST

INTRODUCTION

Today there are sixteen ways to conceive a baby. All of them, of course, use an egg and a sperm, but whose egg, whose sperm, whose conception site, whose gestation site? After the birth of the child, further questions must be answered. Often not even the wisdom of a Solomon can decide who is the mother or who is the father.

Consider a possible situation. If one woman donates an egg that is fertilized in a petri dish and then transplanted into another woman to carry through a pregnancy, is the genetic mother also a mother, or is the birthing mother the only mother? The combinations are many, and the dilemmas even greater. Unfortunately, today little attention is being given to exploring the potential morass of legal, emotional, and societal complexities.

We do not intend to examine the legal ramifications in this book, but where they are germane to a particular issue, they will be mentioned. Disciplines other than ours are more highly trained and experienced in these areas. Our area of focus will be confined to the emotional and psychological effects of donor insemination, as it has an impact upon all of the parties involved.

We wish to emphasize the exploratory nature of this book.

1

It is not intended to be a scientific, statistical study. The nature of the presenting problem, shrouded in secrecy, precluded our ability to design a study that could provide accurate measurements. This does not decrease the work's value; every initial exploration opens doors toward the availability of scientific sampling for future studies. We believe that this is an important study, not only because it presents the problems we found, but because it also presents a point of view and a frame of reference. We came away from our interviews with a strong and clear set of opinions that we will share with our readers.

From February 1980 through December 1982, as part of our formal study, we interviewed people directly connected with donor insemination. These people were interviewed singly, conjointly, and in groups. There was another group consisting of those who either lived too distant to be personally interviewed or who were unable to come to us for other reasons. These we spoke with by telephone at length, and subsequently we received completed questionnaires from them. After the formal study was finished, we continued to meet informally and sporadically with additional individuals, couples, and groups for another three years. We consider the latter groups to be as significant as the study groups themselves because they validated our conclusions and contributed additional important clinical information that enriched our understanding. At the time of this writing, we are continuing to meet with people connected with donor insemination.

A total of 171 individuals took part in the study. Nineteen donor offspring between the ages of 16 and 68 were seen individually and in groups. The majority were young adults between the ages of 20 and 35. One woman was 68 years old. We saw 70 husbands and wives in donor-insemination families. Forty-two of them came from the group in which the husband was sterile. Within that group, we interviewed 12 men and 30 women. Twenty family members came from vasectomied situations; six men were interviewed alone, and seven couples together. All of these people represented

2

second marriages and situations wherein the man had children from a first marriage. Included were four additional couples for whom the vasectomy had been chosen to overcome genetic problems.

Children of these families ranged from infants to 35 years of age. Thirty-one lesbian women in couple relationships were interviewed. Their children were all under the age of eight. Some of the women had older children from previous heterosexual relationships. Fourteen single women who had donor offspring were included in the study. They were between the ages of 34 and 49, and their children ranged from two months to eight years of age. None of these women had children from previous relationships and none had ever been married.

Thirty-seven donors were interviewed for the study. Nine were still actively donating sperm, while 28 had ceased donating between ten and twenty-five years previously. The donors were between the ages of 20 and 50. We did not interview any spouses or children of the known donors.

Our study primarily consisted of individuals from the middle and upper middle-class socioeconomic groups. The only exceptions were within the lesbian groups, where a small number of women came from a working-class background. All of the single women in our study were of exceptionally high-achieving executive caliber and had advanced educational degrees. Most of the donors were either college students planning a medical career or physicians who had donated sperm during their medical-school days; this group was not representative of any large population and was clearly inappropriate for statistical analysis. However, it was, in our judgment, appropriate for clinical evaluation and description.

We hope that other researchers will now broaden our knowledge through more highly scientific studies.

After struggling with the pros and cons of the term AID (Artificial Insemination by Donor), we feel compelled to begin this book by discarding old words and building a new vocabulary. To us, the old language seems archaic and ill-equipped to describe present-day practices. At the risk of courting criticism from other writers and researchers, we propose that the words "artificial insemination by donor," otherwise abbreviated to A I D and spoken as three letters, Ay Eye Dee, rather than as a word, now be changed to "donor insemination," or D I, pronounced as two letters: Dee Eye. DI is shorter, clearer, nonredundant, and more descriptive.

The word "artificial" should be eliminated because it is incorrectly used. It wrongly labels and wrongly describes the procedure. Both sperm and egg are natural and nonartificial. Conception is achieved through the meeting of the fertile egg and sperm, an event also natural and nonartificial. The procedure differs from sexual intercourse because the sperm is ejaculated into a container and introduced into the woman's body manually or mechanically. This difference does not make the insemination artificial.

The combined words, "donor insemination," and the initials DI, are not used in any other field. There is, therefore, little possibility of confusion or misuse of words and concepts. We believe that the terms that naturally follow acceptance of DI as a root expression are also more useful. Donor offspring are the children born of a donor insemination. A donor conception is achieved through the use of donor insemination. The man whose sperm is used in the insemination is a donor father. The amount of money paid to a donor for his sperm is a donor fee. In this book, DI will replace AID, except when quoting another source. We hope that DI will be accepted into the language by our readers and come into normal usage.

Donor insemination has been utilized mainly by couples for whom the cause of infertility is male-related. Sperm obtained through masturbation by a fertile male is placed in the reproductive tract of the woman at the time of her ovulation. We have had close to a century of experience with this type of technology. Brought into existence by researchers in the field of animal husbandry, it is the oldest and most widely practiced alternative method of achieving pregnancy for human beings. The ability to utilize the sperm from one prize bull to produce scores of cattle herds was a boon for ranchers. It is interesting to note that genealogical and medical data for bulls are carefully kept and highly valued as contrasted to human sperm, where records are often destroyed and information denied. For humans, the procedure remains the simplest, least expensive, and most democratic technique. Until recently, DI was principally reserved by the medical profession for the wives of sterile males within a marriage relationship. Women whose husbands had poor genetic histories or had undergone vasectomies were also candidates.

Today, however, we are beginning to see an increasing number of single women and lesbian couples achieving pregnancy through DI. They may choose either to use the traditional medically sanctioned route or to employ a self-help approach, with support from their own networks. They have already changed the prevailing emotional climate and altered opinions by their open attitude. They are challenging old institutions and raising difficult questions.

The donor offspring within nuclear families were not expected to ever learn about their conception. If they did find out, it was usually accidental. It can be assumed that the donor offspring of single women or those coparented in lesbian partnerships will be told of their donor conception. Since most of these children are still too young to provide us with information, we can only try to predict what the emotional effects may be.

The rate of donor insemination has increased steadily year by year, but because of the secrecy practiced by the physicians involved, we have no hard figures on the number of donor offspring in this country. There are many estimates, none of which are reliable, and they are probably lower than the true figures. Donor sperm is readily available; donor insemination is simple to administer. It is not only the specialists in infertility who are able to inseminate patients: Every general practitioner in every small town can easily become an expert. Little thought has been given to reporting the number of cases. In fact, the opposite was and continues to be true: The thought is clearly of *not* reporting or making public the existence of donor-insemination cases in a physician's practice. Records of donors or of women who have conceived through donor insemination are either nonexistent or purposely destroyed.

Occasionally throughout the past decades, negative publicity has surfaced. For example, in a contested divorce, a husband would admit to being sterile and would accuse his wife of having become pregnant without his consent, using donor insemination. The husband would sue his wife to avoid having to support their legal child, insisting that the child was not his genetic offspring. While these cases were few and far between, they made good copy; but they failed to result in widespread discussion or evaluation of donor insemination. They have, however, pointed up the legal confusion and potential problems inherent to the world of DI.

Technological advances in the past decade, beginning with in vitro fertilizations, captured the imagination of the public. They also focused interest on the large number of infertile couples and the need for new methods to help them achieve parenthood. Despite our overpopulation concerns, there was a beginning recognition that the time might come when we would be equally concerned with the high percentage of infertile human adults. All of the potential high-technology methods of conception made news, and the media wrote and spoke extensively about each new development. This finally brought donor insemination out of the closet. In its new form, DI was not only used to impregnate the wife of the sterile partner, but also to impregnate the compassionate fertile woman willing to carry a man's baby for the purpose of giving it to that man's infertile wife. Thus the surrogate mother became part of the parenthood package, raising a whole new generation of dilemmas—ethical, legal, and psychological.

We have chosen case histories as the most readable and clinically accurate way in which to describe the feelings experienced by the various participants in our study. You, the reader, have an opportunity to utilize the information in your own way. We provide you with the story; you provide your own reactions. We are dealing with intense human emotions relating to sexual intimacy, reproductive adequacy, hereditary lineage, parental connections, family dynamics, and many more factors. The need for and the use of donor insemination have a strong impact upon the relationship of the parents to each other as well as to the children. It affects the family as a unit through the secrecy involved and the way in which power is given and taken away.

Each chapter focuses on a different party in the DI picture. Although each story is complete in itself, all of them are connected through our research project. We will acquaint you with the couples who utilized donor insemination. You will follow them through the years and live with them through the many changes in their relationship. You will meet their donor offspring who have learned of their own origins and are living with the knowledge. Donor fathers will tell you their stories, reflecting upon their recruitment as well as their feelings many years later. Nonsterile men who have turned to donor insemination for other reasons are part of this study, as are single women and lesbian couples, whose attitudes and family life with their donor offspring are contrasted with the earlier family stories.

Finally, we want to share our clinical conclusions with our readers. We are strongly in favor of openness and honesty in DI, and we will describe our reasons for this in our summing-up. DI is one small gate into the world of high-technology baby production. If we do not use our experience to date to learn and to modify our attitudes and behavior, we will create greater problems than we can envision. We earnestly hope that this book will contribute toward the growth of sound practices that will build healthy families for future generations.

ANNETTE BARAN
REUBEN PANNOR
Los Angeles, California

"I feel that if
it can't be mine,
then it shouldn't
be her either. . . ."

1 The Genesis of a Study

"**I**f you had your first child through donor insemination, why don't you have your second child in the same way? Why are you applying to adopt this time?"

The social worker looked puzzled. She wondered what information the couple was withholding, and how important it might be.

Ralph and Adeline Mettsintery had hoped that the agency would not raise the question, but here it was. They had to explain their change in direction well enough to satisfy the adoption worker. Adeline looked at her husband, clearly waiting for him to respond. He gave himself a minute to ponder his reply and then plunged in.

"It's more my decision than Adeline's. Adeline liked being pregnant and having Deirdre. You're the first person outside of our doctors who knows that I'm sterile and that Deirdre was conceived through a donor's sperm. I don't mind telling you, because I know that what I say here will be kept confidential. I love my daughter very much, even though she is not mine biologically. I don't love the secret, however, not at all."

Ralph's voice trembled and he struggled to gain control of himself. He continued with great intensity, "I feel that

8

if it can't be mine, then it shouldn't be hers either. We should be equal in this. No more secrets." He paused again and Adeline spoke up.

"I really agree with my husband. I'm glad that I had the opportunity of having one child, and I'm really glad that it was a girl. This time we want a boy, and somehow that makes it even more important that we have this one through adoption. I think it might be even harder on Ralph if he had a son who was really another man's child and everybody thought it was Ralph's."

It is not always possible to identify the germ of an idea for a research project. In this instance, it is. The above interview, which took place almost a decade ago, was indelibly imprinted on the researcher's mind. The words and picture did not surface again until the final stages of writing a book on adoption reunions. While summarizing the need to end secrecy, anonymity, and their resulting emotional problems, suddenly the words, "If it can't be mine, it shouldn't be hers either," rose from some hidden niche. The image of that man, loving his daughter but plagued by secrecy, returned.

The book on adoptions was completed and published, and the plan to research the emotional aspects of donor insemination became a reality. Initially, we expected to study nuclear families with fertile wives and sterile husbands, wherein the children had been conceived through donor sperm. In our simplistic vision, this is where we thought donor insemination began and ended.

We reviewed the literature and found studies pertaining to animal husbandry. There were many articles about the use of prize bulls as studs to increase the value of the herd. There was little about human beings, and virtually nothing about the emotional effect of DI upon the people involved. So we devised our own research design. We settled on a study that would explore the issues rather than measure data from a statistical base. We set about to contact families and interview them. We planned to focus on the feelings and attitudes of women who had been impregnated by donor sperm, the feelings of their infertile husbands, the thinking of the donors, and the effects on any offspring we could locate who had learned the facts of their conception. Since this subject has been shrouded in secrecy, we had to resort to newspaper publicity as a way to recruit participants. The response was greater than we had expected, and our exploratory study was under way.

Because our colleagues expressed great interest, we agreed to discuss the research, preliminary though it was, at a conference. We hoped that other professionals might open our eyes to new directions that we had not yet considered. And they certainly did!

The room was almost full, with only a few seats in the back rows vacant. The audience was largely female, all of them mental-health specialists. This workshop was titled "A Preliminary Exploration Into the Emotional Effects of Donor Insemination Upon the Parties Involved." The presentation covered our project in its beginning phase and raised many issues. When delivery of the prepared material was completed, the researchers asked for questions and discussion from the audience. The meeting was then turned over to the moderator.

A middle-aged woman stood up and began to speak without waiting to be recognized. She looked so nondescript that the contrasting intensity of her tone and phrasing shocked the audience into sudden awareness.

"God, how I wish I were twenty-five years younger! In my thirties, I accepted the fact that I probably would never get married. I came to terms with being single for the rest of my life, but I wanted to have a child then, and I still feel terrible that I never had the opportunity. I feel that I really missed out. I knew nothing about donor insemination, but even if I had known, even if I could have arranged for it, I wouldn't have had the courage. But let me tell you, if I were in my thirties now, I most certainly would have a child by donor insemination."

Finishing on this rather defiant note, she sat down abruptly. There was a moment or two of silence, finally broken by the moderator. With professional aplomb, she thanked the speaker for her courage and honesty and invited others to follow suit with their own feelings on the subject.

Rather hesitantly a hand was raised in one corner of the room. A woman stood up and remained quiet for a moment, in thought. Her tone was soft as she began to speak but gained decibels as she expressed herself with increasing certainty.

"In the fifties and sixties, we women didn't feel that we had many options. I always knew that I had to have children. That's why I got married, and let me assure you, it really is the one and only reason that I did. I can't say that I'm sorry about the marriage, because I did have four kids and I loved the years I spent in raising them. My husband wanted only two children and he was furious when I became pregnant with numbers three and four. I insisted that both were accidents, but I knew so clearly that if I had to have a husband, he had to give me babies. Otherwise, there was no point to the marriage."

From somewhere a voice broke in, "Well, all those babies grew up. Are you still married?"

"You think I am crazy or something? No, I'm not still married. When the children were old enough to be in school all day, I went back to college and started preparing for a single future. I got my degrees and went to work to prove to myself that I could support myself. The moral of my story, I think, is that today I wouldn't have to get married to have children. Maybe I wouldn't have four, but I certainly could have had one or two and raised them as a single parent. DI is a marvelous solution for women like me. It's certainly fairer to the men. I have a lot of guilt over the fact that I used my husband to fulfill my maternal needs. He should have had a wife who wanted to share her life with him, not a wife who suffered his presence because he was her baby-making machine."

The audience was no longer quiet and attentive. People were excitedly talking to one another in pairs or small groups. What had started out to be an academic workshop, research-oriented, had become an emotional catharsis for some that struck a responsive chord in others.

11

The moderator finally achieved a degree of silence and asked if there was anyone present who had indeed become a parent through DI and who was single. Would that person care to share the experience with the group?

There was an instinctive eye-head movement to and fro as the audience looked around, hoping to locate that woman in their midst. They were not disappointed. An air of expectancy moved over the room as a tall, rather commanding-appearing young woman rose from her seat in the first row. She turned to face the audience rather than the podium. With great assurance, she began to speak.

"I would be surprised if I were the only single mother through donor insemination here today. In my experience, these workshops attract people who somehow have a personal as well as a professional investment in the subject. Particularly when the subject is as loaded as this one is. Maybe if I share my experience, some of the others will be more willing to tell you about themselves.

"I have two preliminary thoughts to express before I discuss my DI experience. First, I think this research team is to be congratulated for its interest in this subject, but at the same time, it has blinders on. Why focus only on the nuclear family and ignore single women and lesbian couples? The difference in the different groups' use of artificial insemination is important to study. Secrecy is not the same for unmarried women as it is for married couples. Secrecy is not even the same for single heterosexual women as it is for lesbian couples. Second, I want to express my compassion for the feelings shared by the two women who preceded me. Hearing them talk made me realize how fortunate I am to be able to have my baby my way rather than to have to give up having children, or to have to get married just to have children."

These women, brave enough and forthright enough to speak out, brought a new dimension to our research. They made us recognize the importance of including *all* individuals and groups who utilize donor insemination. We enlarged our study to include single women, lesbian couples, and nuclear families wherein the male had either had a vasectomy or had chosen not to procreate because of a problematic genetic history. Once the dimensions of the study were settled, the task of finding participants and interviewing them began. Since we had no previous studies with which to make comparisons or to enlarge upon, we were really writing upon an empty blackboard.

The more we talked with people involved in DI, and the more we learned about the subject, the stronger our principles and attitudes became. Initially, we had accepted the need for donor anonymity and the inadvisability of telling donor offspring of the truth of their conception. Finally we came to believe that the secrecy of DI was lethal and destructive to the families involved. Additionally, we came to feel that only donors willing to be known to their genetic offspring should be accepted for a DI procedure.

After completing the study, we faced the crucial question: "How should we write the book?" To us, this study was not a compilation of answers on questionnaires. To us, this study was not an analysis of data. Instead, we realized that the true value of our research rested in the people we had come to know and the stories they had told us of their life experiences.

Based upon that recognition, we decided to share those stories with you. Our book, we reasoned, would interest and educate you far more through the words and thoughts of the people themselves than would any distillation we might make of our own.

We chose what we thought were the most representative stories. We hope that you approve of our choices.

2 It Can't Be My Fault

"Everyone just assumed that it had to be her problem. Her parents, Jim's parents, their friends, and most of all, Jim."

Monica had been a little nervous about telling Jim what Dr. Stander had said. She had never expected him to be this upset.

"The hell you say! Just because you got yourself a doctor who's too dumb to figure out what your problem is, he's not going to pass the buck and put the blame on me. No way! Get yourself a new doctor, one who knows his business."

What had started out to be a nice, relaxed dinner was spoiled. Monica knew that nothing she could say now would make it any better. The set look around Jim's mouth and the way he was attacking his food proved it. Still, she had to try to defend herself and Dr. Stander.

"No one's putting any blame on anybody. Dr. Stander simply told me that since all the tests came back normal, he needs a report on you before he can make any definite statements. Part of any complete workup includes the husband. All he wants you to do is to have a sperm test. He needs a check on how many sperm you have and how active they are."

As she described the sperm test, Monica knew that she

was making the situation worse. She was trying to stay calm and to placate Jim, yet there was a part of herself that was becoming enraged. The many months in which she had tried to get pregnant had left her feeling miserable and depressed every time her menstrual period started.

Look at all the months with all those temperature charts, she thought to herself, and all those tests. So what if Jim did have to go and have one test? What was the big deal, anyway? What if it was really Jim's fault, not hers? It would serve him right. Everybody just assumed that it had to be her problem. Her parents, Jim's parents, their friends, and most of all, Jim. They tried to be kind and considerate but she felt as big as an ant with all that "you-poor-little-thing" sympathy.

Jim did not look up from his food while Monica talked. When she fell silent and went back to eating, he put his fork down, raised his head, looked right at her, and said flatly, "Let's get one thing straight: It can't be my fault. Look at me, and look at my family. We're all big and strong. My father, my uncles, my brothers, they have no trouble having kids. We're the first pair on my side of the family to have to work at getting pregnant. You're the first wife in the family who ever had to take her temperature. Now what does that tell you?"

Monica felt like a squashed ant. She was tired of the feeling. Something exploded within her. "Are you afraid to have that test? Are you afraid of what it might show? Maybe you're not the same as your father and your brothers!"

"Don't pull that on me! I'll take that damn sperm test, but I'll make a deal with you. When the test comes back okay, you promise to leave that quack and find a real doctor."

Monica and Jim were shocked at what they had said in anger. They retreated to a safe, neutral place, afraid to risk another confrontation. The subject was delicate, and they didn't know how to talk about it without hurting each other. Neither could figure out just when and how they had arrived at this juncture. Somehow it had crept up on them without their awareness.

* * *

In many ways Monica and James Garthen seemed to be a perfect couple. They appeared to have everything going for them. They had met in their senior year of high school. Jim was captain of the football team, handsome and full of fun. He was an average student, good enough to win an athletic scholarship to the state college. A star in high school, an adequate team player in college, he was not good enough for the pros. He was realistic enough to see that. He knew that he got along well with people and that he could use that ability to earn a living. With the advice and counsel of the coaching staff, he took easy courses, managed to pass them and to graduate from college with a major in business. Among the team's boosters were a number of successful businessmen who were happy to hire graduating players and give them a chance to prove themselves.

Jim was happily settled in a medium-sized manufacturing firm. He was one of the company's best sales representatives, enjoying a good territory and an increasing income. He liked meeting people and selling what he considered was a great product. In many ways he was his own boss and made his own schedule. It was not a boring job because he traveled a little and did not have to follow the same routine daily. He enjoyed the comradeship with the businessmen he called upon and began to think of a number of them as friends. He was still good-looking and prided himself that he had not allowed his muscles to turn soft. He worked out with weights almost daily, and the results were gratifying.

Monica was a few months older than Jim. They had graduated in the same year, but from different schools. They met when she was a cheerleader, rooting for her team against his. From the beginning, Monica and Jim had had fun together. They liked the same zany practical jokes and they laughed a lot. Life was bright and they were rarely serious. There was little that they felt needed to be taken seriously.

Monica was not career-minded. She knew that she wanted to get married, to have children, and to be a homemaker. Instead of college, she chose to take a secretarial course. After all, she wanted to work only until she started a family.

Marrying Jim was a definite goal by the time she graduated from high school, even though Jim did not know it then. They went together for four and a half years and had married right after Jim graduated from college. They had started a joint savings account when they had become officially engaged; they wanted to buy a house as soon as they could, and Monica hadn't minded putting in the lion's share. She was working full time, while Jim had only part-time or summer jobs. Also, Monica reasoned, Jim would be the sole breadwinner after the children were born, so it was fair that she do as much as she could while she was still employed.

Everything fell into place nicely for the Garthens. Life was happy and free of difficult problems. They enjoyed the years of being a young married couple with two incomes and the freedom to take exciting holidays and to participate actively in the social life of their crowd. They bought a little house that would be large enough for the early years of family life. If Jim's income rose quickly, maybe they could move into a larger house in a better neighborhood.

Monica and Jim had achieved their success by planning for the future and living within their plans. They were careful to use a contraceptive to avoid an untimely pregnancy, and they prided themselves on knowing what the future would bring. Sometimes they made critical remarks about friends who complained over finding themselves in unexpected situations. Life for the Garthens did not have unexpected situations. They knew better.

Their plan was to have two children before Monica's thirty-first birthday. They wanted their children to be close in age, and they wanted to be young enough to enjoy their children's activities. They talked about the fun they would have skiing, surfing, hiking, and biking together as a family. Ideally, they would have a boy first and then a girl, but Monica and Jim knew that that was too much to ask for. They would accept whatever they got. However, Jim did say, as a joke, that one of them had better be a boy or Monica would just have to keep on having babies until he got a son. Among their friends the word was out that the way life was going for the Garthens, they would have one boy and one girl, born exactly when planned. The boy would look just like Jim and the girl just like Monica. Didn't they always get exactly what they wanted, when they wanted it?

After their twenty-fifth birthdays, they decided that it was time to plot a pregnancy timetable. The first child should be born within the next two years, preferably in the spring. Spring, they figured, was the best season, because it didn't conflict with Thanksgiving, Christmas, New Year's, and other holidays. With the calendar in front of them, the Garthens mapped out their strategy. Giving themselves enough leeway, they found the months of February, March, April, May, and June acceptable as a potential birthday for their first-born.

The couple took delight in planning the "no-more-birth-control" ceremony. It was a private occasion, just for the two of them; it signified the beginning of a new era. From now on, they would be thinking in terms of a family, of responsibility and obligation. They decided to have an evening of "one last fling" before they settled into maturity and parenthood. First, Monica put her diaphragm, wrapped in tissue paper, into the box Jim held open. Together, they put the lid on and tied a ribbon around it. Jim put it up on the highest shelf of the hall cupboard. Then they went into the living room, where the candles were lit and the game table was covered with an elaborately embroidered cloth— a wedding present, never before used. Jim brought champagne and chilled flutes to the table as Monica served lobster salad on their best china.

It was a special evening, frivolous and romantic, but it brought back memories of being high-school kids overwhelmed with feelings of passion. The only difference was that back in those days, they had been frightened and unprepared for the depth of their emotions. Now they welcomed the passion, and their excitement was more than sexual. Their lovemaking was eager and abandoned. For the first time in years, they made love again and again. They giggled and wondered if they could make a baby that very first night. Wouldn't that be incredible? They felt full of fertility, able to create miracles.

As the months passed without a pregnancy, Monica and Jim could not understand what they were doing wrong. They knew all about the monthly super-fertile period and the prior abstinence from sexual relations so as to make the sperm more potent during those ovulation days. Neither of them had been tense or negative about the outcome, so they could not blame it on psychological factors. Monica's menstrual cycle had always been predictable, and she assumed that she had a normal reproductive system. Jim was a virile man, with a strong sexual appetite. He had never had any trouble in getting and maintaining an erection.

Each of them enjoyed sex and felt that they had a highly satisfactory physical relationship. Before, they had been concerned about not starting a pregnancy. Now that they were ready, why couldn't they "get the show on the road"? During the first few months, they joked about all the years they had used contraception. If they had known how difficult it would be to conceive, they wouldn't have been so careful.

When Monica first called Dr. Stander for an appointment, she did not mention it to Jim. Since it was preliminary and routine, there was no sense in alarming him. He might make her more nervous and anxious than she already was. Dr. Stander was matter-of-fact about the procedures she would be involved in, and very reassuring. He maintained that with her youth, medical history, and good health, she should be pregnant in a short time. Almost as a casual afterthought, he mentioned the possibility of testing Jim later, if necessary.

Monica was so optimistic when she left Dr. Stander's office that she no longer saw any reason to keep her appointment a secret from Jim. Over dinner she confessed that she had begun to worry that there might be something wrong with her. However, now she was sure that there was really nothing to worry about. At the most, Dr. Stander said, it might be a minor problem, easily corrected. Monica told Jim what the medical procedures entailed, but she omitted the part about his being tested. After all, she told herself, it wouldn't be necessary. Why even mention it?

That had been almost a year ago. During the first few months, she had believed that she was in good hands and doing all the proper things to achieve a pregnancy. It became increasingly difficult, however, to maintain a positive attitude. Month after month her body signaled failure, and the doctor's upbeat words sounded progressively hollow to her. She tried not to burden Jim with her misery. After each medical appointment, she figured out something amusing or pleasant to report to him. Hopefully, it would leave him with an optimistic outlook for the coming month.

Maybe the sorriest aspect of this past year was what it had done to their sexual relationship. Sex was no longer a way of expressing feeling. Before their fertility campaign, they would give each other little signals when they felt passionate. Those times had had a special, heightened quality to them as they communicated their desire. All that had slowly disappeared. Sexual intercourse had developed a new language and meaning in their lives. It became a means to conception, practiced at the right times in the right ways to maximize Monica's chances to fertilize her ovum. It was difficult to remember spontaneous lovemaking and how good it felt.

Not that the situation was much better for Jim. He tried not to be short and sarcastic with his wife, but it wasn't easy to control his growing resentment.

"The doctor says that the optimum time for fertilization is Tuesday afternoon. Can you take some time off? I'll arrange my schedule to meet you at home. After that, according to the doctor, we need to have intercourse every day for the next three days."

He felt like a wind-up toy, expected to perform on demand. Luckily, he had no trouble in becoming aroused and carrying the assignment to its conclusion. However, it was getting to be a drag, and he wished that Monica would figure out how to get pregnant and leave him alone for a while. To think that he, Jim Garthen, would ever get to the point of thinking like this!

20

Jim felt that he had done his part; now Monica's asking him to take a sperm test was too much. After that, what else would they come up with? They had already ruined his sex life. Taking a sperm test was pure hogwash. He was a powerful ejaculator; he had as much or more sperm than needed. But when Monica looked so unhappy and tearful, he made himself calm down. God knew, the last thing he wanted was to upset her, which would probably make it even harder for her to get pregnant. Jim told himself sternly to act like a good sport and to go along with this nonsense, if only to make Monica happy.

It really was not as bad as he had expected. The urologist, Harold Dimond, was a nice guy. He took a medical history, examined Jim, and then asked for a specimen. Jim wanted reassurance badly and went into great detail describing his brothers and their children. He was sure that Dr. Dimond agreed with him. He was in such good shape that he certainly couldn't have a fertility problem. It had to be his wife. No question.

So it was surprising to Jim to receive a phone call from the office nurse the following week, requesting another specimen. She said that she did not know the reason, but she reassured Jim that this was not especially unusual. He was a little upset, but he followed instructions and made an appointment to see Dr. Dimond the following week. He was asked to bring his wife along to the meeting.

Jim spent a rather anxious week. Things were not proceeding as he had expected. He kept trying to reassure himself that there was nothing to be concerned about. Imagining the three of them—Monica, Dr. Dimond, and himself—in the office, he visualized the doctor telling Monica that he knew how hard this was on her since he understood how much she wanted a baby. Now he wanted to tell her that she could be absolutely sure that her husband was a perfectly virile man and that she could stop worrying. Jim played the scene repeatedly in his mind, waiting for the appointment day.

The real scene started off just as the imaginary one had, but it soon changed. From the sinking feeling in the pit of his stomach, Jim knew what was coming. Dr. Dimond was being kind and solicitous not toward Monica, but toward him.

As though from a foggy distance, Jim heard the doctor saying, "I had hoped that the first test results were somehow in error and that the second specimen would change the picture. That did not happen. The first- and second-analysis results were the same. I don't know how to soften the picture, because there really isn't any other way to say it except straight out. The truth is that you are sterile, Jim, totally sterile."

Jim was aware that the doctor was looking at him, waiting for a response. He could not meet that expectation, no matter how he tried. Monica reached over and took his hand, but even that felt like a hollow gesture. He was there, but he felt frozen. He tried to remember what the doctor had said. It didn't make any sense.

Then he heard the doctor continue speaking in a quiet voice. The words registered, but their meaning was unclear. Later he would play the dialogue over and sort things out. "I know how hard this is for you to understand, Jim, and I'm sorry to have to give you this news. Although there is no hope, medically speaking, of improving your fertility, there is another alternative. I don't know whether you know anything about donor insemination, but we've been using the process for over half a century to deal with problems such as yours.

"I want to reassure you that our conversation is totally confidential and need not go beyond these four walls. No one ever need know that you're sterile. That's the beauty of donor insemination. We use an anonymous donor, whose sperm will enable Monica to achieve a pregnancy. You and Monica share the pregnancy, and it's exactly the same as if it were your own sperm, because you're there throughout the nine months. You're there during the delivery, and it's your child. You don't deprive Monica of having a child, and since you two will be raising the child together, you will feel exactly like it's your very own.

"Inasmuch as we are extremely careful about our donors,

22

both of you can feel secure in the genetic background. Our donors are usually medical students or graduate students. They're healthy, intelligent, and fine-looking young men. They never know who you are, and you never know who they are. Your child need never know anything about this. Your friends and family need never know. It is your secret."

The doctor seemed satisfied with his lecture. He looked straight at Jim and smiled. "Basically, what I'm saying, Jim, is that it really is nobody else's business."

Monica had a large smile that didn't seem to reach her eyes. In a cheerful, high-pitched tone, she said, "I'm so glad, Dr. Dimond, that you told us about this possibility, and I think it's perfectly wonderful. I totally agree with you that it's nobody's business but Jim's and mine. It really doesn't make any difference whose sperm it is. What matters is having the child."

She turned to Jim and continued. "Of course it will be our baby. We'll go through the pregnancy together, and you'll be with me in the labor and delivery rooms. And then we'll raise the baby together. You are the father and I am the mother. It's not all that important about the sperm. The only important thing is that we'll be a family, the three of us. Isn't that right?"

Jim forced himself to respond. He sounded wooden and unconvincing to himself, but he felt that the words were what his wife wanted to hear and what he wanted to believe. "Dr. Dimond has probably seen hundreds of cases like ours. If he says that they work out a hundred percent, I believe him a hundred percent. I'm sure, Monica, that if you're pregnant and I'm there with you the whole time, it will be just as if it's my baby, too. I want you to be able to have a child, even if I can't make you pregnant."

Monica's smile seemed to relax. She hugged Jim impulsively and then beamed at the doctor, who looked at both of them with a benign, protective expression.

"Let's all agree to keep this confidential. Monica, not even to your mother or to your best friend should you confide one iota of this information. It's best for Jim if no one knows. You must understand, Monica, that it is particularly difficult for a man to learn that he is sterile. Making it public makes it that much harder. Now, why don't you both go home, relax, and talk it over? Get comfortable with the idea. Then, Monica, call me after the weekend and we'll set up an appointment to start the inseminations."

As the Garthens left the office, Dr. Dimond patted Monica on the shoulder. He then turned to Jim, took his arm and looked directly at him, forcing Jim to meet him eye to eye.

"Jim, I guarantee, you're going to be just fine. You're in a state of shock right now. You'll come out of it, and you'll understand that donor insemination is the best solution. It gives you and Monica the ability to have children with no one ever knowing that you're sterile. You'll forget all about the donor insemination once the kids are born. I guarantee you, they will be your kids. Take my word for it."

COMMENTARY

One out of five couples in the United States will face an infertility problem this year. Experts formerly assigned all of the blame to the wife. After all, she was the one who had to become pregnant, maintain the pregnancy, and deliver the baby. Even though we understood the equal importance of sperm and ovum, the husband's responsibility was largely ignored or underestimated. Society and the medical profession conspired to define infertility as the woman's problem. Since the physician was usually a male, he identified with the husband and protected him for as long as possible. The wife also protected her husband and was willing to accept the blame in an effort to keep her husband's sense of masculinity intact.

Wives like Monica accepted the myriad of unpleasant and often traumatic fertility tests as necessary and as an integral part of womanhood. It was their payment for not being able to conceive easily. When the physician had exhausted all medical procedures with his female patient, his request to have the husband brought into the picture was usually couched in apologetic terms. Husbands were asked to undergo a simple medical procedure, but their cooperation was always perceived as a psychological trauma for them.

"He's going to take it hard. Go easy on him. Give him time to get used to it!" were the pleas usually put forth by their wives.

Surprisingly, not only is the woman not always to blame, but current studies indicate that statistically the man carries the responsibility in 40 percent of infertility cases. Thirty percent of infertility rests with the woman, and the remaining 30 percent falls within a gray area of unknown origin or shared responsibility. Infertility is now a worldwide problem, rapidly increasing in scope. Newly identified as a contributing factor is the environmental effect. Pollution, increased radiation in the atmosphere, toxic industrial compounds, excessive exposure to heat, and other modern technological changes are thought to be involved in the decrease of sperm density. If these assumptions are correct, there is even greater reason to be concerned about male infertility.

For most men, sterility is equated with lack of virility, potency, and general masculinity. The infertile man usually feels incomplete and sees himself as different from other men; he has low self-esteem and harbors the profound belief that he has failed his wife in the most important way. In some instances, a man may offer his wife a divorce so that she can find a "whole man," one able to give her children. It should be recalled that in earlier periods, when fertility tests were not available, a wife was often divorced for failure to produce progeny. It was always assumed to be solely her fault.

Although women like Monica are relieved to learn that the problem is not theirs, they do not expect their husbands to apologize for their previous nonsupportive attitudes. Instead, these women feel protective of their husbands' feelings and are eager to be helpful to them in overcoming the trauma as quickly as possible. They feel that they must be supportive to their husbands, and compassionate about the blow they have received.

Physicians such as Dr. Dimond identify closely with their sterile patients. They feel the depth of the wound. Helping the sterile male to find a way for his wife to become pregnant is perceived by the doctor as the remedy for the injury. In the past, even if the man was totally sterile, the doctor might indicate that he would mix the donor's and the husband's sperm so that the husband might think he was the father. Another recommendation was for couples to have sexual intercourse immediately following donor insemination. Although the sterile man knew that he could not produce a conception, he was given a sugar-coated pill to assuage his feelings of inadequacy. It never really worked.

Couples were made aware of other options available to them, such as adoption, acceptance of childlessness, or foster care. However, the choice was often weighted in favor of donor insemination. This gave the wife the opportunity to have a child, and the child would carry half of the couple's genes. Since it was born within the marriage, the husband would feel as though he were the father. He would share in the pregnancy, and no one need know about his sterility. This last point—*no one need know about his sterility*—was the most important element in the man's decision, and potentially the most troublesome.

3 No One Will Ever Know

Carly felt warm and excited all day long. "Tomorrow," she thought to herself, "I will receive the first dose of sperm; it probably won't work this time, but at least we will have started. God, it seems like forever! What a long, dragged-out deal this has been."

It was a busy day in the boutique, with new cruise wear to unpack, press and tag, and fall merchandise to select for early sale racks. Nevertheless, she found time throughout the day to savor her secret, to remind herself that tomorrow would be a special day. She wondered what the young sales-girls would think if they knew that their employer was more concerned at this moment with her ovulation than she was with the exclusive merchandise for which Carly's Closet was known.

Anita, her assistant, knew that Carly had been trying to get pregnant for several years. Anita had always been re-assuring and supportive, and Carly had been glad to have her to share her feelings with, but no longer. As long as Carly had thought that it was simply her own problem, it was all right to talk about it. As soon as the reports had revealed Zack's sterility, Carly had shut up. Zack had been thoroughly depressed and devastated. It seemed somehow

27

disloyal to tell anybody about his condition. Better keep it in Carly's Closet. She giggled at the pun, but from that time on, that was how she had thought about the secret: a secret in Carly's Closet.

Without Anita to confide in, Carly did a lot of talking to herself. As she drove home from the shop in the early evening, her inner monologue ran: "It's really strange when you think about it. Zack never asked me to keep it a secret, and I never offered to. We both just knew that we wouldn't tell anybody. Once we decided on donor insemination, we didn't need to talk about it again. Zack asked me to keep him posted, to let him know what the timetable would be, but that was all. It was almost as if he didn't want to be reminded of his sterility any more than could be helped."

The contrast between their previous openness and their current noncommittal attitude was striking to Carly, and she wondered if Zack was bothered by it. Before they had learned of his sterility, their friends and families had been part of the scene, maybe too much so. Zack had thought it would be better if they simply told the truth—that Carly was slow in conceiving—than have people talking and wondering behind their back. He would tell them that it was just taking a little more time than usual.

If she let herself be honest, Carly had to admit that she had reached the point where she shuddered when Zack began his little public pep talk. Yet she had never asked him to stop. She wondered why. Maybe because she had felt so bad that she wasn't doing what was expected of her— becoming pregnant—that she hadn't felt she had the right to ask anything of him. Now when anyone asked how things were going, Zack shrugged and said something like "still working at it." The way he said it stopped any further conversation.

Carly stopped at the market and picked up some steaks, salad greens, French bread, and red wine so she could make Zack's favorite at-home dinner. "It's funny," she mused. "We each try to make the other feel better, but in such different ways. Zack thinks that if he pats me on the back and announces through a bullhorn that I'm still okay, even though not pregnant, he's doing the right thing toward me. I, on the other hand, put a Band-Aid on my mouth and cook him his favorite foods so he will feel less unhappy. Maybe my way works as poorly for him as his way does for me."

The romantic dinner, with wine and candles, was pleasant enough, and they tried to enjoy the occasion. Carly reminded Zack that she was going to the clinic the following morning for the first "treatment." Zack nodded and said that he knew. When he turned down her invitation to come along, she was relieved. She felt that she had needed to offer but that she would rather go alone, uncertain of exactly why.

Her usual evening ablutions seemed to take on special significance, and she added a few extra routines usually reserved for special evenings out. Like she was single again, going on an exciting date? "What a nut I am!" she giggled.

As she lay back in the tub, she found herself thinking about the man whose sperm she would receive. She knew that he was a student at the university medical school, and that he was healthy, young, and nice-looking, with average coloring and features. The clinic carefully screened its applicants, Carly had been told, to ensure its patients of the best donors possible. Her donor would come to the clinic just a few minutes before she arrived so that the specimen would be fresh, which, it was claimed, assured its potency.

Carly tried to imagine what the donor would look like. She conjured up a picture of a medical-school classroom as the students were filing out. She saw one man after another walking through the door. Each was handsome and young and lean, and each had on suntans and a T-shirt. Finally she stopped at one who had a nice smile and warm, soulful eyes. She chose him to be her donor.

Carly sank farther down into the warm water and continued with her fantasy. It was fun. She followed him to the parking lot and into his little beat-up car, then off the campus and to the apartment he shared with two other medical students. He was sprawled out on the couch, drinking a beer and reading the newspaper, when the phone rang. She heard him talk with the nurse and agree to go to the clinic the next morning.

The scene switched to the next day. He was hurrying out of the apartment building, into his car, and charging off to the clinic. It was still early and the parking lot was almost empty. He rushed into the rear door of the clinic and made his way to the nurse's desk, where he received a wide-necked bottle.

Here Carly faltered in her imaginary photoplay. Until now, she had felt that she knew the proper sequence. But from here on, it was more like guesswork. No matter, she could figure it out. She put him in a small room with a cot, a chair, some magazines, girlie magazines, and a small adjoining toilet. The scene looked reasonable enough.

Now came the important part. Carly shook her head; she realized that she had never seen a male masturbate. She knew that they did, and she knew that that was how her donor's sperm would get into the wide-necked bottle. She knew too that she had fantasized about various men making love to her, but never about masturbating. The scene became disturbing, and then exciting, and then disturbing again; finally he ejaculated into the bottle.

It took a few minutes for Carly to bring herself back into the picture. She moved the next frame into one of the clinic's treatment rooms. She was on the table, her feet in the stirrups, her knees draped with one of those disposable sheets, waiting for the doctor to come in. When he and the nurse entered, she looked up at them . . . and stopped the frame.

"It's only a test tube of sperm," Zack kept reminding himself. "We are a couple, and it's our baby, even though Carly's getting the sperm from a donor. He's anonymous, and he does this for money. It will be our pregnancy and our child, and nobody will ever know otherwise, and it will seem just like everybody else's pregnancies."

Zack had kept up a good front over breakfast that morning. He hadn't wanted Carly to be upset or worried about his feelings. He wasn't clear on exactly what he was feeling anyway. One minute he was up and the next minute he was down. First he shared her delight that the process was finally under way. Then, just a few minutes later, he felt like he had a hunk of lead in the pit of his stomach. Why had he agreed to this business? He should have gone with her so he would know exactly what went on. No, better he hadn't. He probably couldn't have stood it while they put another man's sperm into her.

The morning at the plant moved slowly, even though he had a great deal of work to expedite. As purchasing agent of a medium-sized aircraft-parts manufacturing company, Zack enjoyed a prestigious role, with a good salary and numerous perks. All department requisitions went across his desk before being assigned to the correct purchasing section. At work, he felt quite powerful and important. He had been told that he had risen in the ranks rapidly because he was competent and well-liked. He thought that he had a good self-image and a healthy, strong sense of his own masculinity. At least, if you had asked him about this last month, he would have said that that was the way he felt. Since then, everything had been up in the air. Everything pertaining to Zack had changed drastically. He used to be a man. Now he was . . . half a man, a quarter of a man?

"What good are your balls if they're empty? Without sperm, they're just that—empty!" He had silently raged these words over and over since receiving the death-blow verdict. It had sounded good when the doctor had described donor insemination as a way out of their dilemma. Now Zack wasn't so sure.

He had not told Carly of his doubts, but he had repeatedly gone over the situation in his mind, and he couldn't decide how he really felt. Carly was all for it; she thought that it was good for both of them. She was indescribably happy, and he didn't want to burst her balloon.

Zack prided himself on being an orderly person, with a logical mind. When he could still his anxiety, he constructed a mental ledger with a credit and debit side. He tried to think of all the pluses and minuses of donor insemination. The plus side was far longer than the minus side

31

in number of items. He even wrote them out so he could look at them.

1. Carly gets to have a baby, which she wants desperately.
2. It's easier than adoption.
3. Medically and legally, it's safer than adoption.
4. The donors are smart medical or graduate students.
5. The baby will be our baby, born to us.
6. The baby will feel like mine because I will share the pregnancy with Carly.
7. Everyone will think that I'm the father.
8. Nobody will ever know that I'm sterile.

On the minus side of the sheet there were fewer entries.

1. The baby will have Carly's genes, but not mine.
2. Carly will be pregnant with another man's sperm. She will be carrying another man's baby.
3. The *real* father is a genius with a super IQ. I'm only an ordinary guy, and if the kid takes after *him*, I will feel terrible.
4. I have to start lying when Carly becomes pregnant, and I will have to keep lying for the rest of my life.

"Eight for and four against," Zack counted. "Two to one in favor of donor insemination. The most important thing on the plus side is that it will make Carly happy. I want Carly to have what she wants most in life at this moment: a baby. I can't give it to her: I don't have the equipment. So the only decent thing I can do is to let her get it from a donor. All the reasons I come up with against donor insemination are really selfish and childish. I have to overcome this feeling about another man. Carly won't be cheating on me. She will be lying in a doctor's office, getting a medical treatment. Grow up, Zack!"

Zack shook himself out of his reverie and vowed to quit acting like a baby. He owed it to Carly. She had married him expecting him to be a man in all respects. He had fallen short, and the least he could do was to live up to his commitment. Even if he felt lousy about lying and pretending, it was worth it because he would be making his wife happy. If she was happy, he would be happy. Hell, they both wanted a baby, and this was the only way to have one, so do it they would, and he would shut up now and forever.

It took three months for Carly to conceive. She was patient and relaxed during this time because the doctor had outlined a six-month program of repeated inseminations. Before each new series, Carly found herself reflecting on the donor. It was a fantasy love affair that she played out with her unknown benefactor who carried the secret seed. Replaying the original scenes she had developed before the first insemination, Carly would chide herself and feel vaguely guilty, and unfaithful to Zack. But the imaginary romance was important; it helped her to overcome the cold, mechanical approach to conception. It was so far from the wonderful dreams she and Zack had shared in the moments of their passion. She decided that it was definitely a lousy way to get pregnant. What was important, though, was getting pregnant, no matter how she felt about the way she achieved that pregnancy.

Zack developed his own approach, which seemed to help him. Since it was all in the hands of the doctor and Carly and he was at this point out of the picture, there was nothing for him to do. The best approach was a nonapproach. When the pregnancy was a sure bet, he would take himself out of deep freeze and become the doting husband and father-to-be. Difficult as it might be, he was determined to play his part to the hilt.

For both Carly and Zack, this was a unique time, during which they lived separate emotional lives. They were kind to one another, but remote. Each was involved with a different set of coping problems calling for different solutions.

*   *   *

The announced pregnancy was cause for great celebration within their family and friendship circles. As far as everyone knew, Carly, who had had trouble in conceiving, had finally made it. Carly let them think what they wanted. She was just elated to be pregnant, and Zack found himself easily beaming with joy at her joy. She was like a kid at the circus. Everything and everyone were wonderful. Even her morning sickness was wonderful. Zack was congratulated on all sides. The men snickered and kidded him. At first, when faced with the good-natured sexual innuendos, Zack would tense up and wish he could fade away. But that passed. He could take anything as long as Carly remained happy.

The would-be grandparents were overjoyed. Particularly elated with the news, Zack's father told everyone that he would now have a grandson to carry on the family name. That was not easy for Zack to have to listen to, but he managed. He now added his parents to the list of people to whom the secret donor insemination was bringing happiness. Zack had broad shoulders and a strong back.

The pregnancy was normal and uneventful. Zack did not feel very sexual during this time. He was tender and caring, but making love was far from his desire. He did not examine the reasons for this, but he was adept at convincing Carly that nonintimacy for the time being was in the best interests of the baby. If he had been pressed, Zack might have admitted to himself that it felt wrong to make love to his wife while she was carrying another man's baby. He decided that once the baby was born, he would enjoy reawakened sexual desire for his wife. He told her so, and she was satisfied. The pregnancy was too precious to jeopardize in any way, physical or emotional.

Carly thoroughly enjoyed her pregnancy. She bloomed, and everyone remarked on her beauty and exuberance. What they didn't know was how emotionally filled and excited she was. She had had no idea of how intensely powerful a pregnancy would make her feel.

One evening while dining out with friends, Carly heard

someone say, "Zack, you and Carly make the best-looking pregnant couple I ever saw!"

"What a strange way to put it!" Carly thought to herself. Then: "Ha, little do they know. Pregnant couple, indeed! I'm the only one pregnant, and that's not only because I'm the female. This is *my* baby. I did it myself!"

Zack put his arm around Carly in answer to the compliment. "I may be half of a great couple, but it's all because Carly is the happiest and most beautiful pregnant woman ever. Isn't she marvelous?"

Zack had smiled broadly at his wife and friends and swallowed the rising bile. He wondered what Carly was really thinking.

As the birth date approached, Zack's feelings intensified. Carly wanted him to share in the numerous baby showers, gifts, furniture and layette purchases, name discussions, and so forth. He struggled to keep himself in check; he felt irritated and raw much of the time. Zack was a "junior," and tradition dictated that his first son would carry on the name. He prayed fervently for a girl.

Wanting everything to go perfectly, Carly had completed all of the arrangements, down to the purchase of the cigars for Zack to distribute on the day of the baby's birth. Before they went to the hospital, while Carly was still in the beginning stages of labor, she give him full instructions.

"What a wife I have," Zack told himself. "She can take on the world. She can handle everything by herself."

And Carly did just that. The birth was easy and the baby boy was big, strong, and beautiful, and he was named Zack III. Grandfather, father, and son represented three generations of a family that took great pride in its name and origins. Zack handed out cigars all week long and had his back slapped repeatedly by friends and acquaintances. He brought his wife and son home on the third day after birth. The house was shining and filled with flowers and champagne. Life was beginning for this perfect and happy little family.

COMMENTARY

Most sterile men, like Zack, who utilize donor insemination for their wives, do not deal with the emotional and psychological effects of sterility. They do not give themselves an opportunity to mourn and grieve for the children they will never produce. This process is essential if the sterile man is to overcome his feelings of inadequacy and accept the donor offspring. Most wives of sterile men, like Carly, collude in evading the impact of their husband's sterility upon the marital relationship.

In Chapter 2, our focus was upon the desire of a couple to become parents and the difficulties encountered in achieving a pregnancy. It was pointed out that the emphasis upon the woman's responsibility for pregnancy is still paramount in our society. It is traumatic for the man to discover that he carries the onus, and a cover-up is considered desirable by each partner.

In this chapter, our couple moves rapidly toward that cover-up, without allowing time for exploration or introspection. To the woman, her husband's agreement to pursue donor insemination is total permission to move forward, without the need to think or rethink the decision. After all, she has been seeking conception for a long period of time. Originally, she took the blame; then she shifted it to her husband after learning of his sterility. She joins the doctor in offering donor insemination as the solution. Carly is even willing to let the world still think that the delay has been her fault. In fact, this is usually the time when the secrecy is set into place. To that extent, the sterile man's wife is sensitive to and understanding of the meaning of sterility to her husband. Her goal is to become pregnant and have a baby. Whose sperm facilitates this goal is no longer very important. Even though the process of insemination is cold, mechanical, and without feeling, her goal makes it acceptable to her. When she becomes pregnant, she expects her husband to share her joy and to feel himself adequate as a man now that they are on the road to parenthood.

* * *

During the period when Zack's wife was undergoing monthly inseminations of donor sperm, Zack experienced a myriad of feelings, ranging from anger, despair, fear, and anxiety to withdrawal and depression. He had readily agreed to insemination for his wife when it was offered by the doctor as the obvious solution. He wanted and needed a fast solution because of the depth of his pain. From a mental-health point of view, the opposite is necessary. Zack needed to live with his pain and to experience feelings of loss and grief; he needed to recognize the ramifications of his loss in terms of family name, blood line, genetic continuity, and sense of immortality. Not only did he need to live through that pain and loss, but he needed to recognize how important the shared experience of biological parenting with Carly had been to him. Now not only was he not siring a child, but he and Carly together were not producing the progeny that would have represented their coupling and loving.

In our interviews with sterile men whose wives had had donor offspring, we became increasingly aware of how tentative their feelings about the use of donor insemination really were before the pregnancy was achieved. However doubtful the men may have been, they did not feel capable of changing their minds. To deny their wives the experience of pregnancy was unthinkable for most of them. If they could not provide sperm, they had to let someone else do it for them.

To most of these men, that sperm was emotionally equivalent to infidelity. Intellectually they knew that the sperm came in a test tube and was administered in an impersonal, technical way. However, their gut feelings, based on irrational, illogical considerations, were strong and disturbing. One man we interviewed told us that his feelings had become so intense that he had forced his wife to terminate a donor-inseminated pregnancy. Neither his wife nor the doctor had understood his feelings. The doctor had insisted that he was emotionally disturbed and needed psychiatric treatment. The wife could not begin to identify with his anguish.

Their relationship had deteriorated in the ensuing months and ended in divorce.

The sterile husband with a donor-inseminated pregnant wife faces layers of feelings that rise to the surface regardless of how often they are repressed. The wife is carrying another man's child. The husband has lost his manhood and feels impotent and damaged. The world thinks he is fertile, but he and his wife know otherwise. Their relationship undergoes subtle changes, and the balance of power is shifted.

Much of the man's thinking during the pregnancy is confused and unfocused. Past sexual behavior as well as fantasies reappear and are used to explain his current inadequacy. His present sexual drive is interfered with, particularly in the marital relationship. Some men experience impotency during the pregnancy and avoid sexual contact because they know they will fail. Others need to prove a level of potency and virility and engage in meaningless sexual affairs. They rationalize that they no longer have to worry about getting anyone "in trouble" and that they ought to live life to the hilt. For some of them, their sexual behavior with other women is a projection of rage and anger. They feel that their wife would rather be pregnant by another man than understand and support them. Latent homosexuality may also surface as a guilt-induced phenomenon.

The relationship of the couple can become disfunctional, or at least strained and detached. Usually a wanted pregnancy brings about a sense of happiness and increased closeness for a husband and wife. It is true that even in a planned pregnancy, old feelings may surface to interfere with the relationship. However, in a donor-inseminated pregnancy, the levels of deception and the destructive seeds of secrecy find a fertile field in which to continue developing for a lifetime. Additionally, rather than inducing closeness, the donor insemination separates the couple both physically and emotionally. The woman did not need her husband in order to conceive; it is her solo achievement, and they both know it. With their sexual interaction diminished and their communication on this important matter closed, the relationship is impaired.

Some men and women who have experienced this effect have poignantly described their relationship as silent and sad. On the surface, they say, they pretend successfully and give the appearance of being a happy couple. Under the surface, they say, lies a recognition of the burden of the secret they share. The lie they live begins when the pregnancy is publicly announced; henceforth it is a lie that develops a life of its own.

Carly and Zack and their counterparts all over the world need to understand the importance of open and frank discussion and exploration of their underlying feelings and emotions before proceeding with donor insemination.

4 They're My Children, Not Yours

So, if Marylou felt that the boys were all hers, where did that leave Les? Well, they were a family all right, and Les was the father of the family, but he was not the father in the way that Marylou was the mother.

Whenever you saw the Karnley family together, you had the urge to pose them for a group photograph. They were so wholesomely good-looking. They were nice people, too. In Harvest Heights, the middle-class community where the Karnleys resided, they were well-known and respected. Truthfully, it probably could be said that there were many women who were jealous of Marylou Karnley. She seemed to have everything: an attentive husband, two wonderful sons, a lovely home, a prize-winning thoroughbred dog, a loyal housekeeper. She herself was young-looking at forty-two, with a good figure and a pleasant personality. Her home, decorated in excellent taste, always seemed to be orderly and ready for guests.

If you were one of her neighbors or friends who had rebellious teenagers, a messy house, and a husband who fell asleep in front of the television set, you might wish you could change places with her. How lucky could a person be? Yet, since Marylou was genuinely pleasant and accommodating, it was difficult to resent her success. In fact, she went out of her way to be "old shoe" and down-to-earth with everyone. She could have been snooty and lorded it over the other women, but that wasn't her way.

Marylou would have been surprised to hear all of these things said of her. She was quite unaware of her so-called "perfect image." The only perfect people in her world were her sons, Nick and Jake, and she tried not to let them or anyone else suspect her feelings about them. She didn't want them to be conceited, nor did she like people who bragged about their children. Quietly, but deeply, she enjoyed everything about them. Life was basically satisfying for Marylou, and she felt herself lucky. Once in a while she wondered whether Les, her husband, felt himself as lucky. Was he happy?

"He really should be," she would tell herself. "He has just as much as I do, maybe even more, considering how it could have been."

The Karnleys had just celebrated their twentieth wedding anniversary. Except for one difficult period in their early married life, there had been no great traumas or tragedies. That period had begun when Marylou had become depressed after having tried for almost a year to become pregnant. Finally, after seeing a specialist for months, she was given a clean bill of health. Then when Les was tested, the problem was immediately identified. They were called into the doctor's office and given the verdict.

Marylou's depression was minor compared to the one Les fell into. He could not accept his sterility, and he almost collapsed. It was difficult to believe that her strong, dependable husband could fall apart. He didn't want anyone to know. She had promised not to talk about it—not to her best friend, not to her mother or to her sister—and she had kept that promise. They had made a pact for her to have children through donor insemination, allowing everyone to assume that the children were biologically and genetically hers and Les's.

That bad time had passed as soon as Marylou became pregnant. Les had recovered and acted the role of the proud, macho husband. She had been so glad to have her old husband back that she had put it all out of her mind. Anyway, she had had more important things to think about. Their first child, Nick, was big and beautiful and a delight. After

41

Nick's first birthday, Marylou had told Les that she thought it was time to start on the second baby. He had agreed, and she went back to the same doctor for a second donor-insemination pregnancy. There was no need to talk about the arrangements and the treatments. It was Marylou's business, and Les stayed out of it.

During the second pregnancy, Les again played the proud husband, and Marylou presented him with another big, beautiful son, whom they named Jake. Marylou liked having boys. She didn't care about trying to have a girl. Two boys seemed like a perfect family to her, and she told Les that she thought their family was now complete. Les had agreed. He loved his sons and was a devoted, involved father from the beginning.

If Marylou had asked Les if he was a happy man, he certainly would have answered in the affirmative. He would not even have had to stop and consider. His yes would have been immediate. He had no trouble in counting his blessings. He had a thriving small business, a wonderful wife, and two terrific kids. Compared to others, his life was pretty good. Of course he could recall that unbelievably terrible time when the doctors had told him that he was sterile and that nothing could be done about it. He had thought that his life was ruined and he had almost lost his mind. He couldn't work, he couldn't sleep, he couldn't eat. He had been sure that he would never be happy again.

At night, lying in the dark, Les had considered giving Marylou a divorce so she could marry a "real man." He had even felt suicidal at times. The obvious solution, donor insemination for Marylou, was presented to him at the same time as was the report of his sterility. He didn't hear it then, and he didn't absorb it for several weeks, even though Marylou had kept talking about it. Finally, when he was willing to listen and think, it had made absolute sense. Donor insemination had been his salvation. It had saved his sanity; it had saved his marriage; and especially, it had saved his image before his family and community.

Les was most comfortable when dealing with the "here

and now." He tried not to dwell on the disturbing areas of his life any more than absolutely necessary. "What good does it do to worry if you can't do anything about it?" he would say.

For the most part, he succeeded in living that philosophy, so that he was pleasant and agreeable and optimistic with his friends, his customers, and his family. However, even those who knew him well would have been surprised to know that there was another side to Les. He did a lot of thinking and analyzing, trying to resolve aspects of himself that were confusing to him. He knew, for example, that there was a definite "before" and "after" in his life. He was not the same man he had been before he learned that he was sterile. Maybe no one else could see the difference, but it was there nevertheless, and he knew it deep in his gut. Sometimes he wondered how it would have been if he and Marylou had had the boys together. There was no way that he would ever know. He had had to settle for what he had: a great package, beautifully wrapped, but pretty empty inside.

How could he ever know what a full package would have been like? Les watched other parents and their children, and he particularly watched his brother's family. He wanted to find clues that would help him understand the difference between his family and his brother's. Maybe his brother and sister-in-law didn't have as smart or as well-coordinated children, but it didn't seem to matter to them. Sure, they complimented him on his kids, and they meant it, but he knew that he was missing an important piece that other fathers seemed to have.

He remembered a fishing trip that he, his brother, Mark, and their kids had taken together. In their sleeping bags at night under the stars, the boys had started telling ghost stories. Mark's oldest son, Troy, was holding forth dramatically, and he had the other kids groaning and moaning. The way he talked and the inflections in his voice were so familiar. It took Les back to earlier fishing trips when he and Mark had been in junior high, and about the same age as their kids on this trip. Mark and Troy sounded so much

43

alike. Mark heard it, too. He turned to Les and said with quiet satisfaction, "Listen to that kid, will you! That sounds just like one of my concoctions. Isn't he a chip off the old block?"

Just a little thing, not of any consequence, and yet Mark's words had felt like a sharp knife thrust deep into Les's belly. There was a certain note in Mark's voice, a certain feeling of connection, that Les knew he himself had never had. He wasn't jealous of his brother. Rather, he felt an inconsolable sense of loss; he knew that there were tears waiting behind his eyes.

Another time, at the big summer family picnic, their dad, the children's grandfather, was going through his annual "Karnley kid kount and ketch-up." This was an old tradition in the Karnley family that Les remembered fondly from his childhood. This time, Dad went through the lined-up grandchildren and came to Nick and Jake. He praised them to the hilt, commenting on their physiques and especially on the way they looked him straight in the eye. Then he turned to Les and Marylou, standing off to the side, and said, "Can't get over your boys. It's the damnedest thing. They're the only Karnley males I ever saw who don't have the Karnley nose. Are you sure they're really Karnleys?" He laughed at his own joke, and laughed even harder when one of the cousins said, "They don't know how lucky they are! It's about time somebody escaped that Karnley curse: the Karnley nose!" Les and Marylou had joined in with the humor, but Les had seen the look on Marylou's face. It was like she was saying to his dad, "If you only knew how right you are!"

You wouldn't expect a man like Les to be so introspective. He always seemed to be too busy and too occupied to find time to daydream. The word "volunteer" had been reinvented for Les. He could always be depended upon to come through. If a charity drive needed a chairman, call Les. If a boy's athletic team needed new uniforms or equipment, call Les. He was quiet, but effective and hard-working. Les would tell you that no matter how busy a person was, there was always time for introspection: in bed at night when sleep wouldn't come, while exercising in the morning, in the car driving to and from work, sitting in the stands watching the kids play, and many more. He did not feel that his thoughts were morbid or negative; rather, they were very personal and very helpful. "Mulling around" in his head, as he called it, gave him opportunities to connect with feelings that he hadn't realized were there.

Les had given a lot of thought to the kind of parents he and Marylou were. He had no trouble in categorizing Marylou, because she was a clear case. She was a hundred-and-twenty-percent devoted and loving mother to both Jake and Nick. Although the same might be said about a lot of mothers, Marylou was different in a very basic way. Because of the anonymous donors, Les figured that Marylou felt that those boys were all hers. Maybe she would deny it, but it was true. Moreover, those boys had very super fathers, which made them exceptionally intelligent and special. Marylou didn't really look down on Les, but he couldn't hold a candle in the "smarts department" to the donors, who were probably rich, successful doctors by now.

Marylou sometimes said things that really bothered Les. Because he didn't know how to get her to stop this, he just suffered in silence. She had a little speech that she recited whenever the time seemed appropriate to her. When he heard her start it, he gritted his teeth so hard that his jaw ached for hours afterward. Just last month she had gone into her cute little act again. They had been at Parents' Night at the boys' school. Les was used to hearing the boys praised by their teachers, and he had expected to hear the accolades again that night. The boys' grades were high and they were active in sports and extracurricular programs. A new teacher whom they had just met for the first time was waxing enthusiastic about Nick. Marylou had smiled sweetly and responded right on cue: "You know, I knew when I was pregnant that Nick was going to be very special. You could see that he was smart and intelligent and remarkable from the day he was born." Les had gritted his teeth tighter than ever and thought to himself, "Doesn't she know how that makes me feel? Why can't she just shut up?"

So, if Marylou felt that the boys were all hers, where did that leave Les? Well, they were a family all right, and Les was the father of the family, but he was not the father in the way that Marylou was the mother. He didn't have the same parent power she had. He didn't have the same ownership rights she had. Les knew that these were lousy thoughts, but they accurately described what he perceived. It wasn't even that Marylou was heavy-handed about her proprietary interests. In fact, on the surface she deferred to Les all the time. But her deference had a hollow ring, and Les knew that if he heard it, the boys, who were no dummies, heard it, too.

Les knew that the boys liked him all right and that they compared him favorably to their friends' fathers. Maybe "liked" was the key word. "Liked" was a lukewarm word, and he, unfortunately, had turned into a lukewarm guy and a lukewarm father. He hadn't been lukewarm when he was growing up, and he hadn't been lukewarm when he married Marylou. He had been passionate and hot and intense. Les reflected that, over the years, being sterile had reduced his temperature by many, many degrees.

How did he relate to the boys? It was most interesting for him to try to chart the changes in their relationship over the years. He had been surprised at himself that he had not been overly bothered by their paternity during the pregnancies. Some of the time he had felt like a complete fraud, and he had even tried during each pregnancy to visualize what the donor was like. When he had asked himself how he could handle having his wife carry another man's baby, he could honestly answer that it was better for him this way than not having kids at all.

Although he would have liked to have had girls, Marylou was so delighted with the boys that he had shared her happiness. Girls not of his genetic makeup would have seemed easier to accept somehow. He had imagined himself with a little girl on his lap, or walking down the street holding her hand. It was a tender, affectionate picture. However, Marylou had had two boys instead. He genuinely liked the boys because they were very nice human beings. He was genuinely proud of their various accomplishments. He was glad that they were easygoing, well-behaved kids, because he knew that he would not have been able to be their disciplinarian. This realization was the most confusing of all to him; previously he had not seen himself in this light.

In college, he had signed on as a camp counselor. The university's religious conference sponsored a camp for children from the inner city, and he volunteered for at least one session each summer. The kids who came were tough and street-smart. They tested the counselors up, down, and sideways. Les was one of the few who could resist their manipulations. The kids liked him, but they also respected him because he was strong and could set limits. He was a good disciplinarian, and he enjoyed the role. So when and where had he lost that ability, and why? He just didn't have it anymore.

Had he lost his ability to set limits when he found out that he had no sperm? What a sorry wimp he was if that were true. "Be straight with yourself, Les," he would admonish himself. "Nobody else will hear this conversation but me and me." He finally decided, but not with absolute certainty, that he could probably discipline those kids at camp better than he could his sons. His reasoning went like this: He really didn't have many real rights where Nick and Jake were concerned. How could he feel that he was entitled to lay down the law to those two kids when he wasn't really their father? Their mother, on the other hand, could discipline them without any problem. She had the right to do so. She was for real. He was only for pretend, and pretend took away your moxie.

Actually, if Les were honest with himself, he would have to admit that the family was three on one side and one (himself) on the other. The three were pleasant to him, and tolerant of him, but he wasn't in the inner circle. Or was all of this just in his imagination?

When the boys were little, they were fun. Obviously male, they nevertheless were still rather gender neutral under the large umbrella of children: boys and girls. Lately, however, he had begun to feel vaguely uncomfortable and threatened

47

by their incipient masculinity. They were, at thirteen and fifteen, suddenly developing lower voices and sprouting mustaches. They looked like they were going to be well-developed, virile men in a few years. Whereas he had not been too intimidated by their donor fathers' ability to fertilize Marylou's eggs, now he was feeling hostile toward Nick and Jake's potential to father children. Strange as it might seem, the boys were beginning to make Les acutely remember, and anguish over, his infertility. It was not a subject that he was pleased to dwell upon; he didn't like this part of himself.

Marylou, however, gloried in the boys' burgeoning masculinity. She had always secretly loved being the one woman among her "three men." She had taught the boys to open doors for her, to pull chairs out at the table, and to generally treat her with deference. They had been, from the beginning, her little men; now they were taller than she was. They were emerging with the adult faces and bodies that they would carry throughout the rest of their lives. Marylou took great pride in having borne these boys. More than that, she also carried a connection with their other genetic heritage. They might be known by their legal father's name, but they would be special achievers because of the precious gift of their donor fathers' genes. You could tell, just by looking at them.

Marylou would have described herself and Les as rather average. There was nothing wrong with that, but weren't they lucky that because of Les's sterility and the need to use donor sperm, they had kids a lot more handsome and much smarter than any they would have had together? Oddly, what had appeared to be a family tragedy sixteen years earlier had turned out, from Marylou's point of view, to be a bonus in her life. She hoped that Les felt the same way when he looked at his sons.

Marylou usually ended up sighing heavily after such thoughts. Her sighs reflected sadness that she could not share some of these thoughts with Les. Although she was not certain of what she would say to him, she wished that it were possible to talk about the donor inseminations openly. What made her feel good about them probably made Les feel bad. Did Les ever think about the boys' donor fathers?

Since the boys of course knew nothing of the donor inseminations, neither Les nor Marylou gave any thought to what Jake and Nick might feel if they did know. It didn't make sense to worry about it; Les and Marylou planned to keep the facts of the donor fathers a secret from the boys forever. They saw no value in telling them of their origins now or at a future date.

What about Les and Marylou's relationship? True, they felt that the donor inseminations had protected Les's manhood. True, they felt that the donor-insemination secret protected the boys from the potentially hurtful truth. As a family unit, they functioned well. The boys adored their mother and got along well with their father. What more could you want?

What about themselves as a couple? They were happy together, and they shared many common interests and ideas. They were supportive of each other, and they were genuinely concerned about each other's feelings. Did they each see the relationship in the same light? Did each feel the same way about the family? Probably not, yet both of them knew that they were a fortunate couple. Despite the secret, they could make it. They *had* to make it!

COMMENTARY

Marylou and Les are a good example of a family who guards their secret extremely well. They did not have to fear that their sons would be told of their origins by someone else since no one but they and their physicians knew the truth. In fact, the secret was of such magnitude that they no longer mentioned it between themselves.

During the course of our research project, we met a number of couples similar to Marylou and Les. The media publicity describing our study was read by many people involved with donor insemination. We learned that in some instances, one spouse, after reading an account, would pass it to the other partner without comment. After both had read it, they would discuss the topic for the first time since the conception. Tacitly they would agree to contact us. In other instances, the wife would not feel comfortable about giving the article to her husband. She needed to come in alone initially and then persuade him to talk with us later.

Most of these families were functioning adequately on the surface. They did not consciously know that they were troubled or confused until they read of our research. Only then did they allow themselves to think about many of the unresolved issues that had plagued them for years. It should be understood that they had never considered seeking help. The secret made that impossible.

It was interesting for us to realize how eager many of the women were to discuss these issues. The men, at first loathe to talk about this painful subject, felt vastly relieved at discovering others who understood the meaning of their sterility. The freedom to release inner feelings was enormously beneficial to most of the fathers. These mothers and fathers came forth voluntarily to aid us in gathering data that would not only help themselves, but would benefit other families now and in the future. However, equally important to them was the opportunity, previously unavailable, to deal with secrets that had long festered beneath the surface.

Families of donor insemination do not follow a rigid pattern. In the way that individuals are unique, so are families unique. Nevertheless, it can be said that they do share many common issues. Donor insemination was accepted by the sterile men because it would permit them to appear fertile in the eyes of the outside world. Implicitly, they hoped that they would be able to *feel* nonsterile if they *appeared* nonsterile. If they were *legal* fathers of children, they would feel like *real* fathers of children. But this was a vain hope. The men and their wives knew the truth: The men did not feel the same after learning of their sterility. Even though they kept it a secret, and even though to all outward appearances they had children, they were irrevocably altered in their self-image. Perhaps keeping their situation a secret did much to prevent them from overcoming their feelings of inadequacy. Perhaps they did themselves a great disservice.

For most of the men we interviewed, the choice of donor insemination had been an acute response to the pain they were experiencing. They never permitted themselves the time and opportunity to explore their feelings about the devastating ego blow. They prevented themselves from becoming comfortable with and accepting of their handicap. Instead, they cast the handicap in concrete, and their feelings of inadequacy were continuously reinforced by visual proof: their donor offspring.

With this enormous deficit in place, the relationship between the husband and wife had to be realigned. The husband became weaker and more passive; the wife became stronger and more powerful. The wife was the real mother of the children, and this message, although never spoken, was clearly given to the husband in many ways. The husband could be devoted and caring toward the children, while, at the same time, recognizing the difference between his parental role and his wife's. The children in the donor-insemination family are also aware of the difference in the roles played by their parents.

Although it is true that even in adoptive families, the infertile partner suffers a deficit and knows that he or she is the accountable party, the degree is different. In adoption, both parents are equally not the birth parents. One of them could have been a birth parent, but both chose to equally share in parenting a nonbiologically connected person. In donor insemination, one parent is genetically connected and the other is secretly left out. It is a two-level assault on the husband.

Les is unique among sterile fathers of donor offspring. He is more introspective and self-evaluating than are most people. He acts as his own therapist, and he finds comfort in carrying on an honest dialogue within himself. On the surface, he is mellow and good-natured. He knows that he has lost a good deal of his macho strength, and he has compensated for this loss with other coping devices. Much of the fight has gone out of Les, which is too bad, for he would have been a good candidate for psychotherapy. He has sufficient insight to have been able to mourn and grieve for the children he would never be able to have. He could have accepted himself and probably handled either donor insemination or adoption with a great deal of strength and honesty. He could have maintained a good sense of his masculinity and been a better role model for his boys. Instead, he has paid a high price for his secret, without a good return.

Jake and Nick will probably grow up to be healthy and relatively stable adults, despite the secret in the family. However, they could have had more pluses from their parental relationships had the situation been open and honest. The interactions and undercurrents in a family with profound secrets are slanted and awry. The secret affects all of the members, even though all of them do not know what the secret is or, indeed, that there is a secret. For the children, it is probable that the relationship between their parents, and the way in which each parent relates to them, is subtly confusing.

There are some studies to indicate that donor-insemination families have a lower incidence of divorce than do other families. It has been suggested that they stay together because they are glued by their common secret; if the family falls apart, the secret is in jeopardy. This is an obviously frightening threat to the couple, one to be avoided if at all possible.

In families like the Karnleys, the chances that their marriage will remain intact are extremely high. However, although intact and permanent, there is an emotional erosion over the years. In healthy, non-donor-insemination families, the end of resident parenting can signal a rebirth of early romantic days and a realignment of the marriage relationship that bring with them a renewed closeness and sharing. In the case of the Karnleys, however, the secrecy remains an important element in their relationship, even when the children are grown and no longer in need of protection. It is exceedingly difficult, or virtually impossible, to redefine roles while maintaining secrecy. Donor-insemination couples like the Karnleys carry the secret to their graves. In our study, all of them acknowledged the difficulty of living with this kind of secret, but nevertheless, they could not fathom breaking the pact. At best, the basic kindness and decency of couples like the Karnleys may offer them a frame of reference for building a newly aligned marital relationship at the end of resident parenting.

What would this family be like with psychologically sound ground rules for use as guidelines? How might the couple's feelings about themselves and each other differ? What might the adult children feel if they were to learn the truth of their parentage? If the family is intrinsically sound, we believe it and its component members can not only withstand a new openness, but can indeed become strengthened through new channels of honest interaction.

> "I really think that if a man donates his sperm, he should be willing to have the child he produces meet him. . . . I know that if I ever donate sperm, I will allow myself to be known. . . . I was not conceived by a test tube of sperm, but by a real person."

5 Who Is My Father?

In the sparse literature on donor insemination, there is a notable lack of information gleaned from donor offspring. The reason is obvious: Most donor offspring do not know of their origins. Those who do are not cataloged anywhere in the literature for research purposes. It was important to us to break this silence barrier. How could we recommend an end to secrecy without talking directly with donor offspring? We wanted to know how those who knew the truth had learned it and how they felt about it. How had their feelings impacted upon their family relationships and their own sense of identity? We were interested in the information they had been given and wanted to know if it was sufficient. We wanted to ask them if they felt that openness was beneficial and should be considered in all cases of donor insemination.

Admittedly, we were biased. Our studies of adoptees and birth parents, as reported in our book *The Adoption Triangle*, had led us to the firm conviction that secrets are destructive. We were convinced that there is a direct relationship between the secrets of adoption and the secrets of donor insemination. Without personal contact with donor offspring, our research would be incomplete.

Fortunately, we were able to meet and directly interview individually and in group sessions nineteen donor offspring between the ages of sixteen and thirty-seven. A small sample perhaps, but significant nevertheless. They were located through a variety of means: direct media solicitation, referral from mental-health professionals, and contact with other members of their donor-insemination families.

After individual interviews, we felt that a group session would add an important dimension to our understanding of donor offspring. We were right. Hearing other offspring describe their experiences opened up a deeper well of feeling on the part of the participants. The group meeting was mutually beneficial; we broadened our knowledge, and they gained support from one another.

There were five young people present. We had invited eight, but three were unable or unwilling to attend. Two of the five hesitated and almost backed out but eventually summoned up the courage to come. For all of them, it was an experience without precedent; it was not comparable to any event in their past. Heretofore each of the attendees had felt wrapped in total isolation and had believed himself to be the only donor offspring ever to find out the truth of his origins. So, to be in a room with others in the same boat was truly mind-boggling to them.

Our group was made up of the following individuals:

- Judith (age 28) has an older donor-offspring sister. Judith is the most highly educated in the group, with both a Ph.D. and an M.D. She was raised in an affluent family by whom achievements were measured in material possessions rather than in academic degrees.
- Peggy (age 16) has a younger donor-offspring brother and they live with their divorced mother. The mother works as a legal secretary and struggles to make ends meet. The father is an engineer who provides minimum financial child-support. He visits regularly, accompanied by his girl friend.
- Sean (age 30) is an only child of divorced parents. He is a commercial graphics artist, handsome and poised. Still

single, he is ambitious and talented. Raised by his mother, he has had no contact with his father since his parents' divorce.

- Ted (age 37) is married and has two latency-aged children. He has a younger donor-offspring sister, whom he describes as fragile and extremely emotionally disturbed. His parents have been separated for the past twenty-two years. The father left after his incestual relationship with his daughter was uncovered.
- Bruce (age 21) has two younger donor-offspring brothers. Their mother died four years ago of cancer. Their father owns a garage in their small town and has been trying to keep the family together. He is chronically depressed and drinks heavily. It was during one of his worst drinking bouts that he confided his sterility secret to Bruce. The father suspects that the family doctor is the sperm donor for all three of the boys.

Initially the participants seemed tentative and ill at ease. We began the session (which continued for almost three hours one Saturday afternoon) by describing what we hoped to accomplish at the meeting, and we assured everyone that we would disguise all of the information we received to protect their confidentiality. We also assured them, however, that our motives were to help educate the public on the subject of donor insemination and the feelings of people born from the procedure.

As the tension relaxed, the talk became more spontaneous and the interaction more animated. The following is a summary account of that afternoon; we have attempted to cull the most meaningful parts of the discussion.

Sean was sitting directly to the left of the session leaders. He received the nod to begin telling his story.

- **SEAN:** Being the first to speak is obviously difficult, since I don't know what others will say or what is expected. However, I'm really quite an ordinary guy, so I can't be that different, I guess.

Obviously, my father—that is, my mother's husband when

I was born—was infertile and could not impregnate my mother. Let me back up a bit. My mother came from a rather good family, with pretensions of status and breeding. My father was a first-generation American and ashamed of his background. They were a poor match from the beginning. Although my father agreed to the donor insemination, my mother told me that he was never comfortable about it, and that fact translated through to me. The donor, that is, my genetic father, was a medical student with a physical description that matches my looks. My legal father had a high-school education and worked in construction.

My earliest memories are of an angry home, with harsh words and ugly expressions between my parents. The house was quiet and loving when my mother and I were there alone. Toward the end of the day, when my father was expected home, both she and I tensed up and prepared for the bad hours. My father not only fought with my mother, but he always found fault with me. I tried hard to be a good son, but no matter how hard I tried, nothing worked. I never really knew what I did to make him angry. When I would ask him what I had done, he would say, "If you don't know what's wrong, it's your problem. You should know." Not only the words, but the way he said them and the look on his face were scary to a little boy.

They finally separated when I was fourteen years old. My mother had been quietly preparing for the day when she would feel independent enough to support both of us. She knew that once she left, she could not count on anything from him, and she was right. I, on the other hand, like so many rejected children, kept hoping for a miracle that he would one day wake up and love me and tell me that he was proud of me. It took me years of psychotherapy to resolve a lot of those feelings of worthlessness.

But the beginning of my understanding, and what a relief it was, came with learning the truth of my paternity. I think that my mother was also relieved to be able to take the secret out of the closet. My father moved to an apartment about a mile from our house. My mother went to work as a hospital technician. I had a job delivering newspapers after

57

school. I kept asking my mother when I could go to visit my father. She always put me off, afraid of hurting my feelings. I called my father and left messages on his answering machine. He didn't bother to call me back. My mother could see how unhappy and rejected I was feeling. When I think about it now, as an adult, I realize how much time and worry she must have devoted to her decision to tell me the truth. She had no experts to guide her. She knew only that she wanted to help me feel less rejected.

How did she actually tell me the truth? Very simply and very clearly so that there could be no mistake. She told me that I was a most special person and that she had never had any difficulty with me. Neither had my father, but that wasn't the problem. The problem was that my father could not stand looking at me because every time he did, he was reminded that he was not really my father. He was reminded that he hadn't been able to have any children and that the doctor had found a donor to provide sperm with which to make my mother pregnant.

What made it even worse, according to my mother, was the fact that the doctor had bragged to my parents about how handsome and intelligent my donor father was. That did not make my father feel good, which was what the physician had hoped to do. Quite the contrary. It made my father feel even less worthwhile. Not only was he not a potent man, but he was dumb and ugly to boot.

It didn't make any difference how hard I tried. I could never please my father, and my mother was glad to have him out of our life. She told me to get used to his absence because she didn't think that he would want to continue a relationship with me. Initially, I was shocked, stunned, hurt, abandoned. Slowly it all made sense and I could begin to put some of the pieces together for myself. On the other hand, I no longer had a father, and I tried to think that the donor was my father, but that was hard. For fifteen years I had had an angry, condemning father, and then nothing. My mother was a warm, caring parent, but during my adolescence, when I needed a male role model, I had nothing but two facts: I was the product of sperm that had come from a handsome and intelligent donor, and I would never know that donor, my real father.

Today I have some empathy for that poor man who felt so diminished and inadequate. Now, at the age of thirty, I also feel diminished and inadequate, because half of myself is unknown and will never be knowable. I don't think it's fair. Does anyone else feel the same way?

● **PEGGY:** I guess I'm next. It's really weird, because I'm only sixteen, which is not much older than Sean was when he found out the big secret. And my brother, Jimmy, who is only fourteen, found out even younger. What's a lot different is the way Sean found out and the way Jimmy and I found out. That was the worst! My mother, who was having the biggest fit you can imagine, woke us up practically in the middle of the night. She was so upset, there was no talking to her. She made us get out of bed and sit down at the kitchen table. We were scared that the bomb was going to be dropped, or that somebody had died, or something that bad. It didn't make sense, what she was talking about. And if you think I was confused, Jimmy, who doesn't know anything about sex, didn't know from anything.

Mother kept repeating that it was better that she tell us that our father wasn't really our father, because he was sterile and the doctor had found someone to donate sperm to make both Jimmy and me. She was crying and hugging us, and telling us that she loved us, and saying that it really didn't matter that our father was not our father. You better believe that it was confusing and weird. It's dark and it's scary and Mom isn't making much sense, and we don't know why she's doing what she's doing.

Well, we finally got the whole story out of her over the next few days. It seems that our dad's girl friend, Ellen, and Mother had been having a bad fight. We're used to the fact that Ellen sleeps in the same bed with Dad. It's no big deal to us that she's there all night long on weekends when we stay at Dad's house. I guess we should have kept this from Mom, but we never dreamed she would make such a big deal out of it. It seems that Mom called Ellen to tell her to behave herself better, because she was ruining our morals with her loose behavior. Ellen, you have to know, has one terrible temper, and she doesn't take orders from anybody. She told Mom off and told her that she ought to be grateful that Dad still supported us and took us places because he wasn't our real dad at all. Mom was shocked that Ellen knew the big secret. Ellen told her that she knew everything, that Dad had told her all the secrets, and that Mom had better shut up and keep her cool if she didn't want Ellen blabbing everything to the whole world.

That's why Mom got so panicked that she woke us up in the middle of the night. And of course that wasn't the end of it by a long shot. Dad was really pissed off at Ellen because he hadn't wanted us to know either, but once the word was out, what could he do? He was super nice about everything. He took us out to a fancy restaurant and told us that he loved us as much as if we were out of his own sperm and that since nobody knew whose sperm we had, it was just like it was his. Since nobody but Ellen and the family knew the truth, he was just like our real father.

I've been thinking about this amazing story a lot. I don't think fourteen-year-olds should be told, because they're too young, but sixteen, if you are mature and smart, is old enough. In my case, I think I'm glad that he is not my real father, because in his family, there are bad traits. Like they all wear glasses and have terrible eyesight. They all have bad skin from acne. They get high blood pressure and heart attacks when they get old. So with a donor father, I won't get those terrible things. Maybe later on, I'll think other thoughts. Right now I think I'm okay and that I'm over the worst of it. I sure do want to hear all the other stories, and I'm glad you invited me.

• JUDITH: My story is a bit different, I think. In most donor-insemination families, the man is sterile and ashamed of the fact. My father was not sterile, or at least not aware that he was. In fact, he was quite sure that he was fertile and quite fearful of impregnating someone. He had had a vasectomy in his early twenties, and my mother had known that if she married my father, she would have to have her family through donor insemination or adoption. My father and a long line of his antecedents had familial diabetes, with onset in early childhood. My father had suffered enormously as he was growing up, and he didn't want to inflict that suffering on anyone else. He was really very angry at his father for having been stupid enough to perpetuate his genetic flaws.

Grandfather and Father were at loggerheads about the issue. Grandfather was against the vasectomy, particularly because my father was the only one who could carry on the name. Grandfather came from that old school of martyrs who accepted what God had provided. He did make my father and mother promise never to tell anyone about the donor inseminations. What made that promise so paradoxical is the fact that Grandfather, while exacting vows of secrecy, abrogated the secrecy by his behavior toward my brother and me. He made no bones about treating us like lepers who had no place in his precious, affluent family. We never knew why he didn't like us, and we tried our best to behave and to be polite in his presence. Our parents just shrugged when we asked about it.

Much later, when Grandfather died and the will was being read, we were handed the coup de grace. The other grandchildren were left handsome annuities, trust funds, and heirlooms. The will said tersely, "To Judith and Michael, who carry my son Geoffrey's name, I leave the sum of one thousand dollars each. They do not carry the family genetic inheritance and they are therefore excluded from the family financial inheritance."

Please don't assume that this was the way we learned of being donor offspring. That would have been truly dreadful. It was bad enough that the whole family during that session looked at us with utter disdain. Fortunately for us, the truth of our origins was already an established fact.

As we were growing up, we were well aware of our father's diabetes. He led a rather special life because of his illness. We adjusted to his needs. Some diabetics have it easier than others. My father had a difficult case, often out of control and with the prognosis of greater problems in middle and old age. I am, as you know, a scientist and a physician, both interests probably stemming from my lifelong preoccupation with my father's illness. The more I learned about it, the more concerned I became not only about his future, but about my own. I did not have diabetes, but what of my children? If I didn't have it, what were the chances of my being a carrier? I also knew that many of my paternal relatives had diabetes but that neither my brother nor I had it. Why not? I wondered. It was all very confusing and contradictory, and my parents gave me reassuring but evasive answers that did not satisfy me as I grew older and became more aware. My parents were not evasive people, and their attitude on this subject didn't fit in with their general pattern of behavior.

Finally, when I was a college freshman, I came home from school at Easter break, determined to get to the bottom of the enigma. My father wanted to honor his pledge to his father. However, by that time he was so angry at Grandfather's attitude toward us that the promise was no longer so holy. In addition, his condition had deteriorated, and there was talk of eventual blindness. He desperately wanted us to know that we would never have to face such a situation. So when I brought the subject up again, he was ready, and he told Michael and me the truth.

How did I feel? I felt many different ways in many different layers of my being. I was enormously grateful to this father who had had the foresight and courage to eradicate a line of defective genes. I felt anger at both my mother and my father for having lied to me for so many years so unnecessarily. I felt betrayed by those lies. I also felt rage over the fact that I did not have any way of finding the person who was half responsible for my genetic makeup. I felt grateful to that donor for having given me a good heritage, because I was healthy, intelligent, and well-coordinated. I was also fearful that perhaps I had inherited less-advantageous genes that might show up later in life. I felt, I must admit, somewhat special as well. Here, in this family, I had always felt different. None of my relatives on either side was interested in science or medicine. Now I knew that my interest came not only from my legal father's illness, but also from my donor father, the medical student recruited by the fertility clinic. Michael and I spent a great deal of time talking about this, and I know he felt the same way.

• **BRUCE:** Maybe what is unique about my story is that I think I know who my donor father is. Of course there is no way I can be totally sure, but there is a good chance that my pop is right. He says that the family doctor probably left the examining room and came back with his own specimen to put into my mom's body.

Let me start from the beginning. I'm the oldest of three boys. We're your typical good old American family, living in small-town USA. Pop runs the best garage in town and is a master auto mechanic, and we boys have been fooling around with cars ever since we could bike over to the garage on our own. Everything was fine until Mom got sick with cancer two years ago. Pop and she were really a happy couple, and it just about killed him to watch her suffer. He started drinking toward the end of her life, and he kept it up afterward. He did his best to keep the family going, but he was lonely and depressed, and he would drink himself into a stupor almost every night after he finished his chores. I guess you could call him an alcoholic now, and I'm working on getting him to some of those AA meetings.

Anyway, one night when he was particularly out of it and blubbering away about missing Mom, he blurted out how miserable he had been that he couldn't give Mom babies. He was really crying about how he hoped we boys wouldn't hold it against him that he wasn't our father. He'd got it into his head that he was sort of worthless, and now that Mom was gone, he guessed that we would see right through him and dump him once and for all. I tried to tell him not to worry, but he was so drunk that he didn't hear me, and I finally just put him to bed. He didn't remember anything the next day, but what he had said kept bugging me, so I brought it up again when he was pretty sober and we could talk.

Stan and Brad were with me when we faced Pop, because I figured this was a family matter for all of us to deal with. Enough secrets, I figured. Pop was kind of unstrung that he had let the truth out, but after we told him that he was our pop regardless and that we would never desert him, he calmed down a lot and began to talk.

You have to know about doctors in small towns. Pop said that Doc Braden had been terrific. He took care of all of us, like general practitioners in little towns do. He could set broken legs and deliver babies, and obviously he could inseminate women so they could have babies even if their husbands did have fertility problems. Doc Braden had made the whole thing sound very simple, and he had shrugged off the problem of getting a donor for Mom and told them not to tell anybody about it, because it wasn't anybody else's business.

Pop said that when we kids were growing up, every once in a while he would look at us and catch a glimpse of something familiar. He couldn't put his finger on what it was, but once it hit him that my brother Brad laughed just like Doc did. Pop now believes that we are all Doc's offspring. Pop thinks we are pretty lucky to have Doc's genes, if we can't have his.

God, we three guys would rather have Pop's genes than anybody else's. We don't think of Doc as our father in any way, shape, or form. Pop is our only father. Maybe we would rather not have known about Doc's role at all. But I guess one of the good parts of all this is that now Pop isn't lugging that awful secret around anymore. Maybe the drinking and the misery won't be as bad now that he knows we love him, fertile or not.

● **TED:** Okay, here I am, the last on the program. I've been listening to everybody else, hoping that someone would bring up a problem similar to mine. My story is hard for me to tell. I'm probably the oldest one here today—except for our venerable leaders. I'm thirty-seven and my sister is thirty-five, and we're each a product of donor insemination. I'm now married and I have two children, seven and nine. My family life is pretty good and we are basically happy. However, that doesn't take away the old painful memories and the problems I still have about my mother's donor insemination. For her and for my sister, the effects will last a lifetime, and for me, their pain is my burden to share.

I can't put off telling the facts any longer. We're a Catholic family, and my mother would have loved to have had a dozen children, but my father was totally sterile. So they had two children by donor insemination in the usual secret way. My mother was the kind of woman who believed that you make your bed and you lie in it, no matter what. She was willing to put up with my father's womanizing and to look the other way. She wanted us to respect him, so she always put him in the best light possible. My sister worshiped our father. I use the word "worship" because her love and adoration for him was somewhat overblown and it always bothered me. He and she flirted; everybody thought it was cute. I didn't, and it got worse the older my sister became. Mother resumed her nursing career part-time when both of us were in junior high school. She often worked the evening shift, and I was out a lot with the guys, playing basketball at the neighborhood boys' club.

Now the hard part to tell. I swear I didn't have a clue, but I hold myself responsible that I should have had many clues. If I hadn't been so damn selfish and involved with having a good time with my buddies, maybe I would have caught on that my father was screwing my sister. Now I have said it! If you think I'm consumed with guilt, you don't know my mother. She now accepts the fact that she really knew but that she didn't want to know. If she had faced what was going on, she would have had to do something drastic, and she was too passive and weak to take steps.

My sister tried to tell my mother, who didn't want to talk about it. In desperation, my sister came to me. She had a boyfriend, and she didn't want Father to touch her anymore. Father was threatening her and she was scared. I wanted to kill my father, and I made Mother listen to both of us. I made my mother go with us to the school counselor, and then the law stepped in. There was no turning back. Our family fell apart and has never been the same. That's a laugh. Our family was a phony, shaky house of cards from way, way back. It was during one of those conferences, or hearings, that Mother told both of us that we were not our father's children. I'm not sure whether she thought that would excuse my father or whether it would make us feel better that we didn't carry his sociopathic genes.

If my father thought it was okay to have sex with my sister because she wasn't really his daughter, I don't buy it. She was raised as his daughter, and he should have been able to keep his hands off of her.

Today I feel that I've come through it all pretty well, but like I said, I worry about my mother and my sister.

The group achieved a subtle commonality through opening up their secrets. Leaving their isolation behind, they had achieved membership in the unique world of donor offspring. Even though their life histories differed enormously, the common ground they shared was vast. For the first time in their lives, they had permission to talk freely about having been born out of donor insemination and how they felt about being donor offspring.

We posed questions to the group. Although the participants had previously discussed many of these issues in individual sessions, listening to the reactions of others with similar experiences was important to them, and it gave us further insight into the universal dilemmas inherent to the donor-offspring experience.

QUESTION: *Do you wish there were some way you could find your donor father?*

ANSWER:

BRUCE:
For me, the question is not as important as it may be for others. My brothers and I have a feeling that we know who our donor father is. We don't want to prove ourselves right or wrong. We'll let it be. Maybe, if I am really honest, I have to say that I feel one up on the rest of you, because mine is a more open deal, all the way. I guess that underneath it, since Doc is such a special person in my family and my pop feels pretty good that it is Doc, things are more okay. Remember, Pop feels bad about being sterile, but Pop doesn't feel bad about Doc being our donor father.

PEGGY:
I don't know how Bruce could be satisfied to just "let it be." If I were in his shoes, I would have to find out if Doc were really my father. I would give anything to be able to meet my other father. I wish I could know what he looks like, how he lives, and what he has fun doing. Do I have brothers and sisters out there who look like me? Wow! Wouldn't that be something! You know, what if I met a guy who looked like me and whose father was a doctor? That person could be my brother. What if I fell in love with that person?

JUDITH:
For a sixteen-year-old kid, you are incredible, Peggy. You go right to the heart of the matter. I share Peggy's feelings wholly, but I'm almost twice her age, so I've lost some of my romantic fantasies. Instead, I dwell on harsh realities. Twenty-nine years ago when I was conceived, nobody paid much attention to genetics, recessive characteristics, diseases carried in sperm, and so forth. Now we know a great deal more, and we know how important such information can be.

I'm struck by the difference between adoptees and donor offspring. Adoption records may be sealed, but the possibility of unsealing exists. For us, they made it a point to never keep records. We have questions and no answers. My father and mother were terrific in protecting us from the possibility of inheriting diabetes. Why couldn't they have been terrific in making sure that we could find our donor fathers if we wanted to? I can answer my own question: Everybody was scared of the truth.

SEAN:
Look, I, as much as or maybe more than anyone else here, wish that I could meet my donor father. I really feel that I never had a father, or maybe it's that I never had a father who felt like he was my father. He was there because he had to be, and as soon as he could, he disappeared. If I could meet my donor father, I would probably freak out with fear, but I would meet him anyway. How would my donor father feel? Who knows? Probably just as scared as I would be. I really feel pretty good about the heredity he provided me with, and I think he would be pleased with the kind of person I am.

TED:
Given the lousy father who raised me, you better believe that I would give anything to be able to replace him. However, realistically speaking, I have to accept the fact that my donor father is really only a genetic father. He has no obligation to take care of me or to partake in my life as a meaningful relative. I really think that if a man donates his sperm, he should be willing to have the child he produces meet him. Does that sound out of line? I know that if I ever donate sperm, I will allow myself to be known.

QUESTION: *Should all donor offspring be told the truth? If yes, how and when?*

ANSWER:

JUDITH:
Yes, yes, yes! Look at all of the problems described here today. How much better it would be to know the truth and to grow up with it. I do believe that I always knew something was very different about me in the family setup. Maybe

I'm having mystical hindsight, but I do think that everyone here would agree with me that after they learned the truth, they felt relieved and that things for the first time made sense. Of course, if you open up donor insemination, you must keep records and give parents a great deal of information about the donor parent.

PEGGY:
Don't tell them when they're too young. It will only mix them up. They have to be old enough to understand sex and birth and all that. Maybe people could figure out how to prepare kids to be told later on. Now don't get me wrong. I'm all for knowing, but not before a person can understand.

TED:
I agree with the others, and I would like to add that if a husband had to face the fact that donor insemination would be openly explained to his children, he would have to think the whole process through and deal with his feelings in a different way. Some men might decide that they couldn't go through with it, and that's perfectly all right. Not everybody should have children in this way. I won't speculate on whether my father might have behaved differently if he had not lived with this secret.

BRUCE:
Sure, it would have saved my pop from all that grief. If a man feels that he loves his kids . . . well, that's the most important part of the parent business. Also, Pop saw that all of us felt okay after he told us the truth. It didn't really hurt any of us, and it didn't change our feelings about Pop. And we know that he loved Mom so much that he wanted her to have babies even if he couldn't get her pregnant. It was the damn secret that was the problem.

SEAN:
Bruce is totally right. It is the damn secret that causes the trouble. Look at my family. My father went along with the donor insemination when he probably hated the idea from

day one. Ted said it for me. If my father had known that I would be told, maybe he and I might have had a chance for a better relationship. Of course, there's the chance that I wouldn't exist at all. How about that!

When members of the group were asked for their recommendations, they responded with similar views. To each of them, ending secrecy was paramount, and tied in with this was the need for known donors. They had not been conceived by a test tube of sperm, but by a real person.

COMMENTARY

In other chapters, the interrelationships of people involved with donor insemination have been explored. In this chapter, we have focused on donor offspring.

In the preceding pages, five donor offspring—disguised to protect their confidentiality—have shared their stories with us. Their attitude is representative of the whole group of donor offspring that we were privileged to interview. For us, the experience was unique and exciting in ways we had not foreseen. When our research project was reported in the media, we received letters and phone calls from donor offspring who wanted to tell their history. In addition to volunteering to participate in our study, they wanted to know what we knew about donor insemination, because they knew so little. We were the first people outside of their immediate families whom they had ever told of their origins. Unfortunately, we did not know very much ourselves, because the barrier of secrecy was so strong. We could not tell them, for instance, how other donor offspring felt since we had never met any before this, and because the literature had nothing to offer.

Very soon we learned that all of them shared common concerns. The reason the secrecy barrier had been overcome in their families was not in the interests of openness or honesty; it was not based on any principles, or convictions, or understanding. There was only one reason that donor offspring were told the truth of their paternity: Very simply, the system they lived in had broken down and the practice of secrecy had failed. No one had *planned* to tell the truth. No one had *foreseen* breaches of secrecy. The breakdown of the system was essentially a breakdown of the family, at which time other problems surfaced. In some families, the breakdown could have been foreseen; in others, a crisis erupted, with immediate consequences.

Sean's story illustrates one of the most difficult aspects of donor insemination. When a husband cannot accept his infertility, resents his wife's pregnancy by donor insemination, and is uncomfortable with the child, the seeds of breakdown are sown. Donor offspring such as Sean are constant reminders of their father's inadequacy and failure. Men with low self-esteem and a shaky sense of their masculinity are especially troubled by their offspring, who have been genetically fathered by a virile specimen. Sean, and others like him, must therefore be perceived by these fathers as "bad," imperfect, and lacking in some way, so as to bolster the father's self-image.

The confusion experienced by Sean was alleviated when he was told why his father disliked him so much. However, had he not been told, he might have resorted in the future to negative acting-out behavior in a vain attempt to get any kind of attention from his father. Although Sean is relieved to know that he has not been "bad," his identity search is at a dead end: He has no father, and he has no way of finding his genetic parent or of receiving answers to his questions.

Although the secret may be seen as safe within the nuclear family, when a divorce occurs, the risk of disclosure rises. The father's sterility is never discussed within the family, but outside the family, as a single man, he is no longer thus constrained. The donor-offspring child in a divorce situation is likely to become extremely vulnerable. If his father is distancing himself, the reason for this can be made clear: He is not really the father. If the divorce is bitter, subtle blackmail—in the form of low (if any) child-support payments or the threat of disclosure to the child—is set in place and affects the relationship of the child to both parents. In the donor-insemination family, the mother has great power as the only "real" parent. This position is reversed when a divorce takes place. The mother loses her power through fear that her ex-husband may desert the child, may tell the child the truth, or may publicly broadcast the facts of the child's origins. Donor offspring are inevitably aware of and damaged by these emotionally destructive interactions between their parents.

The incest taboo is clearly weakened in the families of donor insemination, just as it is in step-parent families and adoptive and foster families. While the incidence of incest cannot be scientifically or statistically substantiated, the potential is obviously present, and sufficient evidence exists in the synergistic family to be applicable to the donor-insemination family.

Ted's story is representative. The father, disturbed and emotionally ill, has less incentive to maintain control and structure since he knows that his daughter is another man's child. The rationale that it is "not really incest" because the child is not his is common, and female donor offspring easily become victims when this kind of thinking prevails. Even should the donor-offspring incest victim learn the truth of her paternity, the deep scars are not eradicated; she has been seriously and profoundly abused.

Learning the truth is better than living within the secret parameters of a dysfunctional family, where the problems multiply and fester. However, in donor-insemination situations, the truth does not lead to greater knowledge or to new information. The truth is now juxtaposed against the dead-end barrier of anonymity, before which the donor offspring can only feel further victimized, and powerless.

All donor offspring wish that they could overcome the factor of anonymity. They feel a need to validate their conception by a real person, not by a test tube of sperm. The vacuum in which one half of their heredity has forever disappeared cannot do other than affect them negatively. Their experience differs from that of adoption, or abandonment, or death. In these circumstances, two parents *did* exist, and while they may have been hidden, or buried, or lied about, they were real and identifiable people. In donor insemination, however, the donor is denied existence and relegated to the role of a masturbatory ejaculation, purchased for a third party.

The donor offspring who knows the truth may be relieved to know it, but accompanying this knowledge is the suggestion that he is really only half a person. Nowhere is there a record that would authenticate him. Even in a life-and-death emergency, where knowledge of the genetic father or his whereabouts might save the donor offspring's life, there is no help to be had; all of the bridges have been burned, and the road is closed.

6 I Finally Figured It Out

She couldn't help it. She yelled inside to herself, "You are a product of masturbation, and the guy got paid for it!"

There was no doubt about it. It wasn't even a contest. This had to be the worst day she could remember. Nina wished that it were already tomorrow so the whole experience would be further behind her. Whoever had said that abortions were easy was a liar. She hurt; she couldn't stop sniffling and crying; she couldn't find a comfortable place to huddle into under the covers.

Finally she made herself get out of bed to find the clinic's instruction sheet. Maybe it would tell her what to do to feel better. The envelope surfaced in her shoulder bag and yielded a card and several sheets of paper.

Reading the printout was reassuring. She was experiencing normal post-termination reactions, and she had done all of the right things. Within a few hours her symptoms would diminish. She felt less alone and less frightened; she had the doctor's words to keep her company. For the first time in weeks, Nina found herself smiling. To what dumb low had she sunk that she took comfort and companionship from a photostated list of instructions?

She brewed a cup of strong lemon tea and settled back into bed to study the material from the clinic more carefully. The card was very illuminating. It identified her and

74

gave her a blood type and an rh type. This was the first time she had ever known of her blood type. There it was in black and white, and very official-looking: Nina Blakely, birthdate 1-7-62, blood type AB, rh +.

It was two more pieces of information to add to her personal fact sheet, along with height, weight, and eye color. She lay musing and half-dozing, feeling the onset of vague sensations of relief and relaxation. Knowing your blood type was necessary if you gave or received blood, Nina reasoned, and she probably should keep this information in her wallet in case of an emergency. She tried to recall what she had learned of blood types in her high-school biology class. People got their blood type from the combined blood types of their parents, or something like that. Maybe it was the other way around. More like you couldn't have a certain blood type if your parents had certain blood types. When movie stars were named in paternity suits, an analysis of blood type was one way that the courts decided who was the father of the baby.

Nina dozed off, still thinking of what this blood-type information was all about and what it might mean to her. She awoke with a start to the ringing of the phone. It was dark, and she realized as she picked up the receiver that she had slept through the afternoon and into the evening. Her "Hello" was immediately answered by her mother, who sounded worried. "Nina, you sound half-asleep. Are you sick or something? What are you doing sleeping at this hour? Didn't you go to work today?"

Mrs. Blakely knew nothing about her daughter's abortion, and Nina did not want her to because it would be too upsetting to her parents. Nina had done what she thought she had to do. She could see no reason to involve them when there had been only one answer to her dilemma. She struggled into alertness to convince her mother that all was well.

It was an effort, and she hated to have to lie, but it was better than the third-degree interrogation she would have had to face otherwise. When she put down the receiver after reassuring her mother, she tried to clear her thoughts. The abortion made her think of how she might have been a mother herself, and of how John would have been a father. It was there that the picture split in half. John wouldn't, couldn't, be the father, and so it wouldn't have been anything like when her mother and father had had her.

She shook herself. She and John had been over the matter so many times in the past few weeks. The decision had been made for abortion, and the action taken. It was over, and her family would never know. It would be one more secret in her family, one more secret among the many. She heard her inner voice wondering about the family secrets, and she caught herself. Why was she so sure there were things that her parents had never told her?

Nina had always considered herself the family sleuth, and she still did. To an outsider, the Blakely family would seem to be a normal, average, ordinary group. There were the mother, Gineen, the father, Harris, and the daughters, Nina and Zelda. Each looked very different from the others. The girls did not resemble each other, nor did they look like either parent, but so what? There are lots of families whose members come in a variety of shapes, sizes, and complexions. The looks, she thought, might be one clue, but that was not enough to build a case on.

Nina could not put her feelings into words, but she knew with certainty that there was an unsettled climate in her home. Something was off. In her early teens, when she was starting to try to figure it out, she had decided that she and Zelda must have been adopted; that was the big secret. She had had a good idea, but it didn't hold up. There were photographs taken of their mother when she was pregnant, and there were family stories about each girl's birth. Reluctantly, Nina had discarded the adoption theory, which was too bad because it was the easiest explanation of all. There was also something mysterious and glamorous about being adopted. She could have been a fairy princess, left on the doorstep.

It wasn't as if she did nothing but worry about family secrets. Most of the time she just went about growing up, enjoying her friends, and looking for fun things to do. She hadn't spent much time in wondering about her parents.

However, there was one long stretch when she had sat around the house with a broken leg in a cast; she had been bored. She had watched a lot of television soap operas . . . and she had watched her parents and her sister and herself interacting. It had been almost like having her own family soap opera. All of this had started her to thinking again, and wondering about those secrets.

She had compared her dull family to the exciting ones on the soaps and wondered why, if her folks were so dull, they were hiding some huge, horrendous secret. One of the things she decided was that her mother really was her mother, and her sister's mother, too. If she wasn't their "real" mother, she couldn't be as straight-arrow toward them as she was. If you really thought about it, it was obvious that her father and mother were entirely different as parents. Father was sweet and kind, but when anything heavy happened, he always deferred to Mother. She was the boss lady, no doubt about it. It was as though Father hated to discipline them, or didn't feel as though he had the right to lay down the law. Mother always held the full hand, while Father sort of hung around watching the action.

Nina could remember a few incidents that remained especially puzzling. Although they had happened years before, the images were still vivid. One time Mother had come down hard on both of the girls for bringing home poor report cards. Her lecture had been pretty harsh. She said that she knew their potential and that there was absolutely no excuse for their shoddy performance. By the way she said that she "knew" their potential, she seemed to mean that she knew what she knew. Their father had attempted to lighten the mood by trying to convince Mother that as long as the girls did their best, that was all that really counted. The way Mother had looked at him had somehow been so weird, so strange, so thick with something. Father had stopped in the middle of a word, and then he had abruptly left the room.

And then there was another incident that took place when her parents were arguing about money. Mother had wanted to spend more than Father had thought they could afford.

Nina couldn't recall what the money was to be used for: it had to do with the girls and something Mother wanted for them. She did remember, however, with total recall, her mother putting an end to the argument. How she did it was so abrupt and decisive that it had taken Nina's breath away. Father was being very logical and reasonable about their expenses when Mother suddenly erupted.

"Enough now!" she had cut in, almost hissing. That shut Father up, and she looked straight through him. After a few seconds, she continued. "You know very well that in the end, if I've made up my mind, you'll find the money. That's all there is to it. It's for me to decide what my girls need. You really don't have the final say, and you know it."

Nina had felt sorry for her father and was angry at her mother for treating him so badly. Using these clues, she had come up with the romantic idea that maybe Father wasn't really their father. Maybe Mother had had two passionate love affairs and become pregnant by her lovers. Maybe Father knew the truth but he loved Mother so much that he was willing to accept her cheating; he wanted her under any conditions.

This fantasy fit in with the exciting sexual stories of the soaps, and she had nursed and embellished it for a few days. Then, although she tried hard to picture her mother in this mold, it didn't work very well. First, maybe there could have been one love affair and one pregnancy, but two? Second, Mother came from a family and a time when women were fairly prudish. It was difficult to imagine her as an unfaithful wife, meeting a lover in a motel for a steamy afternoon. Nina was back at square one, with no new clues. She had still believed that there was something strange in her family, but since she did not have any other leads, she had given up trying to figure it out.

She had not consciously considered the family mystery for years. But now, keeping the abortion a secret from her parents and trying to keep herself from becoming maudlin over it, she was once more playing mental games with the old enigma.

The years away from home—living at the university and

becoming weaned from the family—had changed her attitude, she thought. Gaining emotional and financial independence, and living as an emancipated single adult with a successful career, should have detached her from the family and its secrets . . . but the desire to solve the mystery was still strong within her. Perhaps her psychotherapy had prepared her for the reawakening of this interest. Under counseling, she had learned more about herself and had developed new insights into the relationships within her family. She realized that she was again enjoying the prospect of reevaluating her origins.

She had a sudden moment of clarity . . . she could at last find the words with which to describe the relationship between her parents. It was as if Mother held something over Father's head. Mother knew something about him, or herself in relation to him, that made her more powerful than he. In all those years when Nina was growing up and playing Nancy Drew, it was the parenting roles that had created the unsettled climate.

If it wasn't adoption and it wasn't illegitimacy or infidelity, what else could it be? If her father wasn't her father, could he be sterile? Could she and Zelda be her mother's children but not her father's? If he was sterile, possibly her mother had been inseminated. That procedure could certainly be used in two separate pregnancies.

Her mind reeled with this new line of thought. For the first time, she had an idea that seemed plausible. Nina felt that her head was full of jigsaw-puzzle pieces waiting to be put together. Where to start? How to make order and logic out of the jumble? She was no longer a romantic teenager yearning for a soap-opera existence. She saw herself now as a capable, intelligent adult, able to correlate information and achieve a resolution.

Jolted out of her reverie by a sharp cramp, Nina came back to the abortion, and she suddenly remembered the card with her blood type written on it. Maybe it was totally out of whack to use this as a positive, but if the abortion were to help her, however indirectly, to solve her personal mystery, the experience wouldn't have been all bad. If blood tests were used in courts of law to determine parentage, why couldn't she use a similar method? Both of her parents had had medical procedures and surgeries; they had to have known blood types. Maybe it wouldn't lead to anything conclusive, but on the other hand, maybe it would, and it was certainly worth a try.

Nina instructed herself to approach her plans slowly and judiciously, and to be patient. If she had already waited for twenty-four years, she could give herself a little more time. Before she did anything major, she had to have all of the facts in place and be pretty sure of the validity of her conclusions. She did not want to look like a fool. More important, she did not want to hurt her parents' feelings, or disturb her relationship with them.

In the months that followed, Nina surprised herself with her patience. She continued on a slow but sure path to gather data with which to prove her hunch that both she and Zelda were donor offspring. Since it was a personal quest, she decided not to involve Zelda yet. Maybe later, maybe never.

Years later Nina would recall the months after her abortion as a unique period in her life. The relationship with John was history, and she was not ready to trust anyone else. Focusing on her genetic origins (as she came to think of her project) gave her a sense of direction. Her social life was almost at a zero. In the past, during times of nonromantic involvement, she and her unattached women friends would become closer and share more confidences. However, this time it was different. Nina was not comfortable in discussing her suspicions of being a donor offspring; perhaps she feared her friends' disbelief and scorn. She felt herself to be different and special, like a CIA agent on a secret mission, collecting clues. This kind of thinking made her giggle to herself; she was behaving like a little kid, but nevertheless, it was the way she felt.

Nina set herself a number of tasks that she pursued diligently. To learn as much about the world of donor insemination as possible became a priority. Unfortunately, the library at the local university yielded little literature, but she learned what she could. None of the articles made her doubt her hypothesis. In fact, the reverse occurred, and she became even more firmly convinced of it. As she read about sterile men and their fertile wives, memories were triggered. She could clearly hear her mother saying that bearing a child was a woman's greatest experience. Her mother always expressed great compassion for women who could not have their own babies. If her mother felt that way, it followed that she would have been heartbroken at the news of her husband's sterility. For her father, agreeing to donor insemination for his wife meant giving her a precious gift and assuring her of happiness and fulfillment. The more Nina thought of these things, the more likely it seemed to her that she might be a donor offspring.

Her second priority was more difficult. There was no scarcity of information; here the problem was technical. Nina lacked the scientific grounding to understand the data on blood types and subtypes. She finally accepted her limitations and checked out a high-school biology textbook from the library. The chapter on blood types was basic and very readable. Even more important, Nina's blood type, AB, was perfect for her purposes. If she was correct in her conclusions, an AB required two AB parents, or one A parent and one B parent, or one AB parent and one A or B parent. Neither parent could be an O type. More specifically, for Nina that meant that if her father were O, he could not be her genetic father.

Her third priority required thinking and plotting. What she now needed to complete her dossier were her parents' blood types. Since she was already certain about her mother, the question rested with her father. If she were lucky, her father would be an O type and the question would be settled. The information she wanted was in their internist's files. How to get it? What to say to convince the office nurse to give it to her? Not that she was asking for any confidential data, but what if the nurse became suspicious and then called her parents and aroused their concern? If Nina described herself, the oldest daughter, as currently making a folder for each parent to have in case of emergency, particularly when traveling, it might make good sense to the nurse. Nina rehearsed the story, and it made good sense to her. If she were the nurse, she would believe it, and as a matter of fact, Nina decided that she would indeed make such folders.

When the project was all over and Nina knew that her father was an O type, she realized how very easy it had been to gather the information and to develop her case. Now the difficult part was to find the courage to confront the situation and face her parents. She toyed with shelving the whole thing. She had the facts; the mystery was solved. At least one part of it was. She knew that her father could not be her genetic parent, and she was almost certain that she was the child of her mother and a donor. Why not leave it alone? Why disrupt her parents' lives? Who would benefit? Who would suffer? While all of this was mulling around in her mind, she made each of them a folder. They went off on an art museum tour prepared for medical emergencies, and Nina did not consciously think about her donor status during their absence.

The day after her parents returned, she found herself sitting with them in their den. There was a lull in the conversation, and without forethought, Nina heard herself tell her mother and father what she knew. She spoke simply, to the point, and without emotion. She would have said, if asked, that she knew without the shadow of a doubt that she was a donor offspring. However, suddenly and much to her bewilderment, she needed confirmation from her parents.

Her mother and father seemed momentarily frozen in the midst of motion, unable to talk or move. The room was very quiet. Finally her father stood up and turned toward the hall leading to the master bedroom. Nina and her mother rose and followed him. Nobody said anything. Once in the bedroom, Nina and her mother sat down on the queen-sized bed and her father shut the door behind them. He sat down on the dressing-table chair and faced them.

"You're right," he began, "and I'm sorry. You see, I couldn't have children but I wanted your mother to have them, so the doctor found donors for you and Zelda. I don't know how you figured it out, because I was so sure that neither of you girls would ever know."

Nina heard the quietly spoken, self-effacing words. She couldn't help it. She yelled inside to herself, "You are a product of masturbation, and the guy got paid for it!"

Nina had her confirmation of the truth given to her by her father behind the tightly closed doors of the bedroom. There was no one in the house but she and her parents. Was his admission still a secret, one to be kept from the walls of the rest of the house? While she sat there, trying to quiet her inner turmoil, her father began to talk again, this time more confidently.

"You know, I'm surprised at myself, but I am really relieved that you know and that it's not a secret anymore. I have felt bad all my life that you and Zelda weren't my true daughters. I felt sad that I couldn't have fathered you, but I love you both very much. I don't know how I would have felt had I been your real father, because I'll never be able to have that experience. I do know that you are the only daughters I have and that I am so glad that I am your father."

Then Nina heard her mother crying, and she realized that she herself was crying, too. Her mother's crying seemed all right to her, but when she saw the tears streaming down her father's cheeks, she almost panicked before reaching out to him. Then, the two of them, Nina and her father, were holding on, hugging each other.

"It's all right, Daddy, it's all right. It will be better from now on. I love you, too."

COMMENTARY

Nina, it must be admitted, is a rare individual; she is unusually intuitive and perceptive. More important, she is tenacious. Although there are few people with Nina's persistent drive, feelings similar to hers run throughout the lives of donor offspring.

It is important to understand that the cornerstone of all donor-insemination families is *secrecy*. Families who live with deep secrets develop a system of interpersonal relationships and power positions that differs from that of ordinary families. In secret-bearing families, many clear but unspoken messages pass between members. Because the secret is tightly held by both parents but never shared with the children, the inherently unequal balance in the parenting equation is subtly and imperceptibly sensed by the offspring.

In adoptive families, if the adoption is kept a secret from the child, both parents fear lest the child be told the truth by an outside source. Adoption is, after all, a known phenomenon in which neither parent is genetically involved with the child's existence. However, in donor insemination, one parent, the mother, is the known and visible parent of the child. The father is the pretend parent who, with his wife, shares the burden of the secret. In both adoption and donor insemination, at least one parent is handicapped because of infertility. In adoption, the parents achieve a degree of parity by choosing to parent a child born of two other people. In donor insemination, the parents choose to permit the mother to conceive and to bear the child of another man. The mother, therefore, feels more powerful as the "real" parent in the family.

In donor-insemination families, the children feel the subtle differences in parental roles, even though they do not know the reasons for these differences. Nina knew that she had a strong, powerful mother. She had many fantasies during her childhood and adolescence about her origins, trying to organize her confusion and bewilderment. Simply, Nina lived in a family where the mother had title to the children, and the father knew it. When he appeared to ignore that reality, the mother reinforced her ownership quickly and unmistakably.

Nina was afraid of confronting her parents with the truth, because she had lived her whole life outside of truth. As a member of the family, she was a participant, unwittingly, in the perpetuation of the secret. In all of the situations we have seen where donor offspring learn the truth, no matter the way in which they learn it, the result is finally a relief for everyone. The fear is over. The only negative fact remaining is that the biological father, i.e., the donor, is unknown and unknowable. The inability to know one's genetic origin leaves a void that deprives one of a sense of wholeness.

7 If I Knew Then What I Know Now

Dr. Phil Simmons looked forward to a free, easy weekend. His associate was on call and there were no really sick patients to worry about. At forty-eight, Phil could and did pat himself on the back frequently; he was a successful physician, specializing in internal medicine. He had an agreeable wife, and two kids who performed well and were destined to do what was expected of them. He felt young and fit and played a good game of tennis. He lived in a beautiful house in a good neighborhood and drove a new imported sports car. Life was terrific, and at four o'clock on Friday afternoon, there was only one patient conference left before his weekend began.

He did not know what Gerald Berg wanted to discuss with him. Berg had been a patient of his for several years, but at thirty-one, he came in annually for his physical examination and little else. Phil tried to remember significant details of their last contact, almost eight months ago, but nothing came to mind. He shrugged and pushed the button, signaling his receptionist to bring Berg into his office.

There was a good rapport between the two men, and they greeted each other casually but warmly. Gerald Berg was a big bear of a man with a ready wit and a comfortable man-

86

ner. He was a businessman, given to straight thinking and talking, without guile or introspection. He clearly respected Dr. Simmons but was not intimidated by him.

Today, Phil noted, Gerald seemed somewhat subdued and troubled. Without waiting for the usual small talk and opening banter, Gerald launched into a monologue that seemed to be well-organized and summarized, as though carefully thought out and prepared for this meeting. No response was expected of Phil, and he sat back to listen, pleased that his patient trusted him enough to ask for the consultation.

Gerald Berg and his wife, Melinda, had been together for six years. They had lived together for two years before marrying. They had carefully practiced birth control until about two years ago, when they had felt emotionally and financially ready for parenthood. Each of them came from a fairly large family, and they had had no reason to worry about their ability to have children. During the first year of trying to achieve a pregnancy, they had rationalized that they were in no hurry and that nature could take its time.

Melinda was the first to begin to voice concern. All of their friends were starting families. Why couldn't she get pregnant? Gerald tried to be reassuring, but he was beginning to feel anxious himself; maybe there was something wrong with Melinda. He agreed that she should consult an expert in the field.

Gerald was not a scientist, but he had learned all that he could, and he was able to describe to Dr. Simmons the various tests, procedures, and medications that Melinda had been given, the lack of positive results, and the effect that all of this had had on her. Melinda had been a fairly happy, spontaneous woman, but after months of living by a temperature chart and a calendar for sexual behavior, she had begun to slip into a dulled emotional state.

Gerald had tried to be supportive and to reassure his wife that their love was not dependent upon her ability to bear children, but his efforts hadn't helped much. Finally the fertility specialist felt that he had thoroughly investigated Melinda's situation and that it was time to bring Gerald into the picture. Until that time, Gerald had never considered that he could be part of the problem. Not that it was not logical to examine both of them, but he was a healthy, virile man without symptoms of sexual inadequacy.

Gerald had not tried to protect himself, nor had he rationalized his feelings of discomfort and anxiety at the results of his fertility evaluation. He had been brutal and self-accusatory, and now he was clearly asking for help and support from Dr. Simmons. When the urologist had somberly revealed that Gerald was aspermatic and therefore sterile, Gerald was unprepared for the blow inflicted upon his whole person. He could not believe the test results and had attacked the physician's competency. He had sought a second opinion, and the results were the same. The second physician had been blunt and had held out no hope for a reversal of the sterility. Gerald was ashamed of the effect that this was having on his feelings of self-esteem and on his manhood.

Although the second doctor had had no medical remedies to offer for Gerald's condition, he had offered hope to the couple in the guise of donor insemination, which he had been practicing for many years with great success. The confidentiality he guaranteed meant that no outsider would ever know about Gerald's sterility. Gerald, the urologist assured him, would feel exactly as though the child were his own. The donors were first-rate physical and intellectual specimens, culled from the ranks of medical and graduate students.

The situation had been difficult for Gerald to integrate into any semblance of comfortable reality. What, he wanted to know, did Dr. Simmons know about donor insemination? How did sterile men feel about their wives being impregnated by another man's sperm? And what about the donors? Did Dr. Simmons know any men who had been or were now donors? What were they like? Why did they do it?

At the beginning of the monologue, Phil Simmons had been relaxed and attentive, wanting to help his patient with whatever problem he might present. As the story unfolded, Phil's composure left him and he felt himself struggling to retain a professional demeanor. He knew a lot about donors, and because what he knew was disturbing to him, he rarely thought about donor insemination. He knew so much on the subject because he himself had been one of those super physical and intellectual specimens recruited by a fertility clinic.

Phil realized that Gerald had been looking quizzically at him, waiting for a response, and he brought himself back to the present. He nodded to Gerald, cleared his throat, and put on a thoughtful expression while he composed himself to answer as a professional, not as an old-time donor. He heard himself explaining the medical facts and procedures and describing the professional competence of the physicians involved. Then he brought the conference to a rather abrupt close by suggesting that Gerald give himself time to become accustomed to the situation; they would arrange to meet again in two weeks for further exploration of the issues facing both Melinda and Gerald. Gerald was grateful for Phil's concern and interest; he did not seem aware of the physician's discomfort.

As he waited for the traffic to clear at the driveway of the parking lot, Phil gave himself a strong message: "Come on now, you've got a free, relaxed weekend ahead of you. Put the office away! Forget Gerald Berg."

He turned the radio on to listen to the news as he maneuvered the car through the late-afternoon traffic. But images and scenes came unbidden into his mental window, and he realized that he had blocked out the radio voices with his inner dialogue. He was back in 1960, a skinny, intense freshman in medical school, talking to a senior over a cup of coffee. Dr. Simmons punched the radio button off and gave himself over to remembering Phil Simmons, one of the most successful sperm donors in his class.

He could picture the other guy, but he couldn't remember his name. He had been cool and matter-of-fact about being a donor. "Hell, man, there's nothing much to it. They give you all the rules on a written sheet. You make fifty dollars a week for a few minutes of work; you can't really call it work, because you jack yourself off for free anyway. This way, you save it to get paid for it. The reason I'm suggesting it to you is that they're looking for new donors in the new freshman class, and you fit the bill. They want guys who are average—

not too tall, not too dark or too light, not too big- or too small-boned. They want uniform facial features. It all pretty much describes you. You're a very average type of guy, and for this project, that makes you a number-one choice."

Phil had been flattered, embarrassed, and broke. He did not know if he could masturbate and ejaculate on command, but if he could earn fifty dollars a week, he would try almost anything. Without making a commitment, he had agreed to think about being a donor and to meet with the clinic director to discuss it further.

During the next few days, Phil had gone through a roller-coaster ride of feelings. Sitting in the student lounge, he had been tempted to talk about the "recruitment" with fellow students. He rehearsed asking offhandedly, "Any of you guys been approached about donating sperm?" but he couldn't say the words aloud. He couldn't figure out whether he was ashamed or whether he felt like bragging. Maybe he felt so special that he didn't want anybody else to have the honor? Maybe he was afraid that he would be looked at as some kind of weird sex machine? Maybe people would be offended on religious or moral grounds?

Since he talked to no one about being a donor, he continued to talk to himself and to try to analyze the pros and cons. On the pro side there was the money, which he could use, no question of that. Also, there was no question but that he was flattered at being identified as a good specimen: virile, masculine, healthy. Idealistically viewed, it was simply a way of helping infertile couples become a family, and that surely was a positive. Nothing wrong with that. On the con side of the ledger, there was only a vague feeling of discomfort, which he could not quite come to grips with. Going to a clinic, getting a bottle, and entering a cubicle to masturbate was not very appealing, but it also was not a terrible thing to do, and it wouldn't take long or ruin his day or keep him from studying.

By the time the clinic director's secretary called to set up an appointment, Phil had convinced himself that he was a fortunate guy and had decided that if they would hire him, he would accept the job and act as a sperm donor as often as they would permit, providing he got paid every time he appeared on their doorstep. For the present, he did not need to advertise his new part-time job, but after he became experienced and comfortable with it, there was no reason to keep it a secret. Donating sperm was a perfectly acceptable occupation, and moreover, it was a helping thing to do.

The fertility clinic was housed in a modern medical building, occupying most of the fourth floor. Dr. Brandston was running late because of an emergency, the pleasant receptionist informed Phil. However, as soon as he had settled himself with a magazine in the waiting room, a nurse appeared at his elbow with a manila envelope. The envelope had his name on it and contained a packet of papers. There were questionnaires as well as information sheets, and he busied himself reading through the material. It was an impressive assortment, with a great deal of factual data, most of it about the clinic and its operations. He assumed that this was the same information given to couples referred to the clinic for donor insemination.

He was still busy with the papers when Dr. Brandston came to the waiting room to invite him into the inner office. It was a nice personal touch, and Phil was aware of feeling rather special. Dr. Brandston treated him like a colleague, explaining the clinic's operation and its staff and welcoming his questions. Phil was reassured of a continuing involvement with the clinic. Dr. Brandston made him feel like a member of a very select club, chosen for special physical and mental attributes. The doctor endorsed donor insemination as a solution to the loneliness and misery of the infertile couple. Phil, Dr. Brandston explained, could make the difference between a fulfilled, happy family life for a couple and a bitter, empty, childless existence for that same man and woman. Without Phil, the couple might well divorce or live a life of frustration.

Dr. Brandston settled back into his large leather chair and moved into the second phase of the interview, now that he had convinced Phil to join the ranks of donors. A medical history was next on the agenda. He asked Phil about his family's history of illness, his own history of childhood diseases, and then rather apologetically brought up the subject of drugs and alcohol. He did not delve any further when Phil explained that he used neither. Each agreed that social drinking was acceptable.

The final test and the most important, Dr. Brandston announced, was a sperm test, needed to check the sperm count and motility. He smiled as he finished with the statement that he knew without a shadow of a doubt that Phil would pass with flying colors. He handed Phil an instruction sheet to cover any unanswered questions. The most important fact to remember, Dr. Brandston advised, was to abstain from sex or masturbation for three days prior to donating sperm. In that way, the clinic could be sure of a rich specimen that had a good chance of achieving a conception.

Phil nodded thoughtfully to all of the information, determined to be the best donor that the clinic had ever had. After he went through his first test, producing a specimen that tested high and healthy, he shook hands with the doctor and the nurse and left in great spirits, eager for his first assignment.

He was still elated when the phone call came a few days later, summoning him for his first donation. It was an early morning appointment. The office nurse was still setting up her schedule when Phil arrived. She handed him a bottle and showed him to a small room containing a cot. Several "girlie" magazines were available on a lamp table standing at a corner of the cot. He giggled softly and then admonished himself to behave like a professional.

The traffic light turned red and Phil came to a full stop, returning to this late Friday afternoon more than twenty-five years later. He shrugged and shook his head slowly. What he remembered so clearly was receiving a phone call from Dr. Brandston himself in relation to that first donation. Dr. Brandston had congratulated him and informed him that he had struck gold on his first try. The woman was pregnant, and both she and her husband were ecstatic.

After that, the months and the years had passed without any memorable donor events. He usually donated twice a week. It became a routine process, and he thought little of it. Just another job that meant he could take his girl friends out to dinner and to a show and that he was a little less dependent on his family for his expenses. He rarely saw Dr. Brandston, and he rarely checked on the results of his donations. In fact, he rarely thought about the consequences of his clinical masturbation.

Throughout his student years, he was conscious of holding to the rules of the clinic. This was sometimes a drag, particularly when he was passionately involved with a new woman. Sometimes he would explain the need to put off lovemaking for three days because of an appointment at the fertility clinic. Nobody seemed to be very interested. In fact, if anything, it was a source of kidding and joking.

But there was more kidding, often with a lascivious touch, at the boardinghouse where he lived. The regular sperm donors were referred to as "the studs," but it was all good-natured banter and Phil felt that the other students envied him his easy source of income.

He remembered only one uncomfortable occasion connected with being a donor. It was during a vacation period at the end of his freshman year, and he was at home visiting his parents. They were finishing dinner, and his mother asked him about his finances. His parents were surprised that he had asked for so little money. They gave him a gentle little lecture about appreciating his concern over their financial situation. Perhaps he was carrying his concern too far. How was he able to manage on so little? They knew that he could not work and keep up his grades.

Although he had not planned to tell them, he found himself grinning and bragging about the easy money he was earning by donating his sperm. He described how he had been recruited and implied that it was something of an honor to be accepted by the fertility clinic. He had expected his parents to respond with excited pleasure at this coup, and he was taken aback by their silence. After a few moments, he asked them why they looked so strange. What was bothering them? They were broad-minded; what didn't they like about his being a donor?

Neither of them at that moment could put their discomfort and disapproval into words. Both his mother and father felt that somehow they wished he hadn't started donating or that he would stop. Later that evening, his mother came into his room and sat down on his bed. She had a look of discovery on her face. She had finally figured out what was bothering her about his being a donor.

"Philly, it's not just your sperm you're selling. Those are my grandchildren you are making, and I won't ever see any of them or know who they are."

They had laughed together at her words, but his mother was not really joking. Underneath, she was serious. He told her that he disagreed with her and that he planned to continue because he thought it was not only okay to do so, but because he thought it a worthwhile role he could play in helping infertile couples.

Today he thought about that sperm and all of his mother's grandchildren, the results of his donations. He shook his head, sighed, and clucked aloud. He felt like an automaton, but he couldn't help it. It was as if someone had wound him up and he was reeling out a lot of unthought-of thoughts. He was not agitated or upset. On the contrary, he was very controlled and determined. He needed to organize his thoughts logically in order to understand that young medical student and to relate himself in the 1960s to himself in the 1980s.

Having been a donor and getting paid for it was not too hard for him to accept. But all of those children out there that he had fathered were a helluva lot harder to deal with. What kind of an idiot was he to have donated his sperm without feeling responsible for the children who would be born with his genes and his looks and his brains and his . . . . What kind of a macho stud got satisfaction from being told that he had the best sperm in the community? And what if his son or daughter married one of his offspring?

He realized that the control he was trying to maintain was slipping away and that his emotions were taking over. Perhaps it would be better to review the donor period in a more factual way. How many years had he continued to work for the clinic? How many times had he donated? How many children had he fathered during that time? Even if he could not come up with the exact figures, he certainly could approximate the numbers. Three hundred? Four hundred? More?

Phil had driven this route daily for so many years that he could put himself on automatic pilot. However, he suddenly realized that he was nearing home. It was time to bring himself back to the present and to his family. Later he would retrieve those questions and find some answers, or at least come up with more questions that might lead to some answers.

It was a busy, people-oriented weekend, and Phil had little time for quiet thinking. But he could not avoid a feeling of disquiet and anxiety when he was with the children. He found himself looking at them intently. He felt as though he were looking at their faces with new eyeglasses that brought their features into sharper focus. These two children carried his name, but there were others whom he now had to consider and come to an acceptance of having sired.

During the following weeks, Phil settled into a phase of greater serenity, with less acute discomfort. He called several fertility clinics to acquaint himself with their procedures. He was doing this in preparation for his next appointment with Gerald Berg, he told himself. He learned that anonymity was still the rule in donor insemination and that there was no way in which anyone could identify the donor now or in the future. He learned that the pay scale for donors had risen somewhat and that medical and graduate students were still the donors of choice.

Increasingly, Phil realized that he had to come to grips with the knowledge that he might have dozens of genetic offspring living right in his own community. They could never find him and he could never find them, nor would he want to. Whether *they* would want to find him was another question, but since it was a dead-end street, why worry about it? He vaguely promised himself that when his children were ready to marry, he would carefully observe their potential partners. If he had any inkling, even the most remote, that there was something genetically familiar about the proposed candidate, he would research it further. In the end, he reassured himself, that was the only real worry he had.

From one of the fertility clinics he had contacted, he had learned of a research project on the emotional aspects of donor insemination. He wrote to the sponsors, offering to participate and to share his feelings about having been a donor. He somehow felt a little better by breaking silence in a way that might be meaningful for others.

Phil prided himself on being a moral and ethical human being. He had tried to fit the donor role into his life framework, with little success. He had to content himself with the realization that he wished he had never been recruited to be a donor. He wished that they had found him unacceptable (but that he had had good sperm as well). He wished that he had not been so eager for money, or that he had been mature enough to refuse the offer. He wished that he had had the foresight to know that one day twenty-five years later he would regret that period in his life. But there was nothing to be done about it now. The past was past. If his son was ever recruited and asked his opinion, he would surely advise him to turn the offer down. If his son asked his opinion . . . if his son followed his advice. . . .

COMMENTARY

Phil Simmons is a typical donor. Initially, as a young student, he saw no relationship between his sperm and biological fatherhood. He did not consciously perceive the consequences incurred as a result of donor insemination.

Unmarried, still emotionally an adolescent, the typical donor has no understanding of the emotional impact of fatherhood, nor of the feelings that reproducing himself genetically will bring in later years. The young donor has little room for introspection and empathy. He is not concerned with the meaning of donor insemination for all of the people involved. He cannot conceive of the lifelong implications of his actions, either for himself or for others.

In its simplest form, donor insemination is a business transaction. Phil became a vendor, offering a product for which there was a demand. He sold his product for an agreed-upon sum to a buyer. The protection and anonymity serve as by-products that further trivialize the meaning of the trans-action to the donor. His responsibility ends with his deliv-ery of the sperm, he believes. In Phil's case, he was approached by a fellow student who acted as a recruiter for the buyer. College newspapers often run ads like the following:

> If you are a healthy, intelligent male, 18 to 35 years old, with a good sperm count, we need you. Become a paid sperm donor.

The response to such ads is generally greater than the need. Student donors feel that it is a good part-time way to earn money. Fertility clinicians are not concerned with donor motivation as long as the donor is healthy and good-looking. There is a small group of donors who believe in their genetic superiority and donate in order to spread their progeny across the human landscape.

In large city medical centers, the recruitment and selec-tion of donors entail a sophisticated and technical effort. However, in every practitioner's office in every small town, donor sperm is present and easily available. There is some evidence that in the early years of this century, doctors themselves acted as donors for their patients. They would excuse themselves from the examining room, produce a specimen, and return to inseminate the patient with the freshest product. Of course, neither the patient nor the hus-band was aware of the identity of the donor. The doctor believed in all honesty that he was providing a necessary service to his patients and that he was acting in a human-itarian manner. From a technical point of view, donor in-semination is extremely simple to perform. It does not need expert administrators or high-tech equipment.

In retrospect, Phil Simmons, the father, has a very different feeling about his donor activities than did Phil Simmons, the student. He is typical of the physicians we interviewed who had been sperm donors during their medical-school days. The parent-child relationships awaken in the ex-donors a sense of regret, concern, and fear for those other children whom they fathered without any recognition of their fatherhood. Many of them see that person in that period of their lives as irresponsible and immoral. They have additional concerns that their offspring might unknowingly marry one another; certainly their socioeconomic worlds may be similar.

There is no accurate information about the genetic, congenital, or communicable diseases that were transmitted through donated sperm in past years. However, there is now ample evidence that diseases such as hepatitis, acquired immune deficiency syndrome, gonorrhea, herpes, syphilis, vaginitis, a type of pneumonia, and chlamydia can be transmitted through donor insemination. This evidence creates a climate in which the type of screening and the extent of testing of the donor must be greatly elaborated. Currently there is some question concerning the continued use of fresh sperm versus frozen specimens. Because fresh sperm must be utilized within a few hours, insufficient time is provided for sensitive screening.

In essence, being a sperm donor is not a role to assume without grave consideration. There is responsibility connected with the genetic transference between the donor and his biological offspring. It is a lifelong responsibility that should not be secret and anonymous. Just as we are now responding to new dangers in transmitted diseases, we must also respond to new awareness of the emotional and psychological effects of sperm-donation as it is now practiced.

"Not many men are
as thoughtful and
concerned about
their responsibility
in reproduction."

8 My Genes Should Not Be Reproduced

E van was the youngest male of a venerable lineage. The Foglers were old stock that could trace their heritage for eleven generations. In the United States, such lengthy historical evidence of family background is rare. Not only was the name, with all of its European spelling variations, available for documentation, but the achievements and contributions of each generation were also recorded for posterity. Evan's mother's family, the Masters, could not account for as many generations, but it was equal in almost every other respect. Evan took take great pride in his forefathers, for they had been physicians, professors, lawyers, and government leaders. Evan, his father and his grandfather were physicians. From his earliest memory, he had known that he would be a doctor. He had not deviated from his dedication, and he had achieved his goal surely and quickly.

Evan had received another contribution from his ancestry, inherited childhood diabetes. He had learned at a very young age to live within the confines of his illness and to restrict his life accordingly. His diabetes was often out of control during his early childhood, and he was a very sick and frightened child.

"Now, when I think back on my childhood, I realize how

difficult it was for me. Then, I knew no different. I grew up with daily urine tests, shots, food that was weighed on scales, and a mother who tried hard to be calm but always looked tense and worried. I learned to be an expert on my symptoms and to ward off dangerous consequences with rapid treatment. If I suddenly felt weak or dizzy, I knew I needed an orange for quick sugar. I knew what I could do and what I couldn't do. Mainly, I knew what I couldn't do that other kids could. I could join the Boy Scouts, but I couldn't go camping with them, or on cookouts. I could play on teams, but the coaches were admonished to keep me from too much exertion. I could invite kids to sleep overnight at my house, but I could never sleep at their houses."

Evan exhibited a great deal of compassion for that little boy, and admiration that he had handled himself as well as he did. It was as if he were talking about someone other than himself, someone whom he was viewing from afar.

"I know that a lot of kids balk at being sent to summer camp. I was the opposite. I wanted so much to be able to label all my clothes with my name and pack them in a duffle bag. I had visions of myself on the trail with a backpack on, and a tin cup hung on my belt. The notion of spending the night under the stars in a sleeping bag seemed so romantic to me as I was growing up.

"Diabetic children are never accepted in regular camps because of their medical problems. My parents knew how much I wanted the camping experience, and they felt so bad for me. My mother did something quite remarkable, I think. She decided that if I felt this way, there must be other diabetic children who shared the same deprivation. So she enlisted the help of a group of doctors who specialized in problems of childhood diabetes. She offered to do all the spadework if they would back her. She set up a special summer camp for diabetic children, with doctors and nurses in attendance. Using an existing nonprofit camp, she started with one session the first year and eventually went to two sessions. Every summer for over twenty years, over a hundred diabetic children have been able to enjoy between two and four weeks of camping and nature study. The camp still exists and is enormously successful. What a wonderful experience that was for me and for other boys and girls like me."

Suddenly the detachment was gone. Evan was sharing some very deep memories that had shaped his thinking. Here was a man who looked to be strong and in control of his feelings. Underneath, however, lay a mass of emotion, channeled into positive action with much effort after long years of anguish.

"I went through a variety of emotional roller-coaster rides throughout my growing-up years. Certainly I have to admit that there are a lot of secondary gains derived from being a sick child. You don't have to be a genius to recognize the attention and special treatment available almost at the drop of a hat. On the other hand, when I wasn't being a spoiled brat, I was often in a great rage at the unfair hand I had been dealt. Or I was angry at my parents for having produced me, with my serious defects. I wished I had never been born. I made them feel guilty, I'm sure, when, as a teenager, I yelled and screamed that I would never want to bring a diabetic child into the world. I've since learned to be glad that I was born and that I am alive. However, I still don't want to ever bring a child into the world with my genes."

Evan is probably in the top one percent of the population in terms of intelligence. He is thoroughly knowledgeable about his illness and the possibility of further medical problems later in life. He knows that he can try to avoid some of the potential hazards by careful medical monitoring and a healthful life-style. However, he also knows that some of the problems of diabetes are out of his control. But he does have control over whether or not he reproduces his defective genes. He knows that the chance of passing the diabetes on to his children is very great. In his evaluation, he would be irresponsible if he knowingly presented a child of his with his own fate. He describes such behavior as criminal.

Family pride, status, and belief in generational connections become unimportant when compared to passing on diabetes. Since he expected to provide his child with a smart, nondiabetic medical-student donor father, Evan was not worried about sacrificing IQ points. Even if he were, he would rather have an average-IQ, healthy child without diabetes; he would rather have a below-average-IQ child without diabetes. He would rather have no children than risk having one with diabetes. That was how strong he felt about passing his illness on to anyone else.

Since he did not believe that there would be any great advances in curing diabetes, or in isolating the responsible gene, during his lifetime, he decided to undergo a vasectomy while still a medical student. His parents were sad about it, but the strength of his conviction closed off any further consideration. To him, it was a nonnegotiable decision.

It was not easy to find a physician willing to perform a vasectomy on a twenty-two-year-old man. It was a procedure too final and irrevocable. How could Evan be sure he wouldn't be sorry later for this "rash" decision? Evan did not feel that a decision reached after twenty-two years of living with a terrible disease was in any sense "rash." He was sure, and he finally found a physician who concurred with his right to have the procedure performed.

Although Evan had had a few semi-serious relationships during college and medical school, none of them had made him consider relinquishing his bachelorhood. When he met Maureen in his senior year of residency, he was ready for marriage, and she seemed ideal to him. Maureen was an oncology nurse, compassionate but detached with her patients. Not so toward Evan. With him, she let down her outward reserve, and he responded with passion and tenderness.

From the beginning of their relationship, he was honest with her about his illness and his vasectomy. He wanted to marry her, but he knew that she might not want to deal with the problems he presented. He wanted to parent children with her, even though he would not be their biological father. He wanted to have a family . . . if she could see herself using donor insemination. If the idea of a donor pregnancy was anathema to her, he was willing to adopt, but he really preferred children born to her.

When you spend years thinking through a problem to find a workable solution, as Evan did, you can present a very convincing argument. To Maureen, this was new and uncharted territory, and she did not know what to think or how to feel. It seemed somewhat bizarre and confusing. In the final analysis, however, she decided that above all, she loved Evan and wanted to spend her life with him. All other decisions followed from that recognition. Maureen had grown up planning to get married and have children. Evan was the husband of her dreams, and she wanted to have his babies, conceived out of their love for one another. Now she was having to adjust to a new set of parameters, to make the rearing more important than the having of the children.

"Of course I don't want to have sick babies, or babies with a chronic medical condition," she told herself. "Of course, from choice, I would prefer to have normal, healthy children. Evan is absolutely right in his decision to avoid the possibility of passing his diabetes on to the next generation. Not many men are as thoughtful and concerned about their responsibility in reproduction. That's one of the special parts of Evan. He has had to overcome so much in growing up with severe diabetes, and he knows that he doesn't want to see a child of his repeat that experience. The more I think about his decision to have a vasectomy, the more I appreciate the wisdom that went into it, and the more I love him. Of course I would rather conceive a child through making love to the man I love. I absolutely hate the idea of getting pregnant on the examining table, but I'll survive it, and we'll share the pregnancy. It will be our baby, because we'll know why and how we made our decision."

Although Maureen and Evan were private people, they did not view their use of donor insemination as a deep, dark secret. Most people, strangers and acquaintances, would never know about Evan's diabetes and his vasectomy; it was none of their business. On the other hand, there were a number of people close to them whose business it truly was, and they deserved to know the truth. The children they would have were, of course, number one on that list. Grandparents were right behind, and then close friends.

As it turned out, it was especially important to tell Maureen's parents the truth. They were very upset at the thought of their daughter marrying a diabetic and bringing diabetic children into the world. It was bad enough that Evan might someday be blind or crippled or amputated and that Maureen might have to take care of an invalid in later years. It was worse to think of the children suffering from very the beginning of their lives. They were against the marriage until they learned that Maureen planned to use donor insemination.

Evan had no sympathy with men who knowingly continued to reproduce hereditary or familial diseases. As a scientist, he understood that often the presence of such problems could not be identified until after the birth of the first child. For example, he had a colleague whose first child was born with Tay Sachs disease. No one in either family, as far as the couple knew, had had the condition. However, both families were first-generation Americans, from eastern Europe, and Jewish, factors closely associated with the disease. It was heartbreaking to watch the tragedy within that family. The baby was not diagnosed until he was over six months old, and then he began to deteriorate day by day. They tried to care for him at home but finally had to institutionalize him. In the meantime, the couple received genetic counseling and learned a great deal about recessive genes and Tay Sachs disease. They were told that there was a 25-percent chance of having another Tay Sachs baby.

Evan identified closely with the couple and assumed that they would not try to have any more of their own children. He took it for granted that they would either use a donor or adopt a child. He was aghast when they blithely went on having children. They had one more Tay Sachs baby and one normal baby. Today he finds it hard to be friendly with this colleague; he considers the man to be selfish, irresponsible, and stupid.

Within a year and a half after the wedding, Maureen gave birth to a healthy little girl. Two years later, a baby boy joined the family. Both of the children looked like their pretty mother and her side of the family. Maureen and Evan still lived in the university community, and they had tried to use the medical-school clinic for their inseminations.

Once Maureen had accepted the idea of donor insemination, she became an avid proponent of as much openness and interaction with the donor as possible. She was instrumental in convincing Evan that they should meet the donor and get to know him. It was not difficult for Evan to go along with his wife, because he had no unresolved infertility issues to cloud the picture.

Naively, they approached the director of the medical-school fertility center with their request. After much discussion, Maureen and Evan had arrived at a "laundry list" of their needs. They asked to meet the donor and to get to know him through a series of informal meetings. They wanted the same donor for two children. His promise to inform them of any medical problems that might affect the children's health was important to them. Probably most crucial was an agreement that the donor would be available to meet his offspring when they reached a reasonable age.

The center director was adamantly opposed to every item on their list. He tried to assume an amusing and flippant attitude toward them, but the discussion soon disintegrated into a hostile argument. Maureen and Evan were upset that they were not taken seriously and that their feelings were discounted. Finally, in an attempt to close the breach, the director tried to explain that the center policy was one of total anonymity and that no exceptions were ever permitted. He further indicated that he felt they needed to rethink their position.

Undaunted, they did a little research on the other members of the center staff and chose one of the associates, Dr. Frank, as potentially more approachable. In addition, Dr. Frank had a private practice, which was not subject to the rules of the fertility center. It was not easy to win over Dr. Frank, but Maureen and Evan argued their case convincingly and intrigued the doctor with the thought of an open insemination. He viewed it as an experiment and began to consider possible donors. Grant, a regular donor in his private practice, had expressed interest in meeting the couples who would raise his offspring. He seemed to be a good choice.

Maureen, Evan, and Grant met on four occasions before

beginning the insemination process. Initially tentative and diffident, they soon relaxed and realized that they liked each other and had much in common. Were they not assuming their specific roles, they might have become friends. Grant was in total agreement with Evan's vasectomy decision. He felt that using a donor under such circumstances made sense. He shared with them information about himself, his family, his background, and his life-style. As Maureen said, "If I can't have you, Evan, for the genetic father of my children, Grant is a superb second choice."

Although Maureen and Evan had not made specific arrangements for Grant to see the child, a meeting came about quite naturally and easily at the time of the insemination for their second child. Evan was sitting with the baby in the automobile in front of Dr. Frank's office, waiting for Maureen. As Grant left the building, he recognized Evan and came over to say hello. Both men were self-conscious and embarrassed for a few moments. No etiquette book covered this kind of meeting. When Evan jokingly acknowledged this, the ice was broken. Grant smiled and shook his head in wonderment. "What a special surprise! How wonderful! This is a first for me and for you, and for this terrific kid. He's big and beautiful, and he looks just like Maureen!"
Evan responded with delight and generosity. "He's truly a remarkable child, and of course I'm not the least prejudiced. I think he looks a little like you, particularly around the eyes. Don't you agree?"
Evan smiled and continued, "You did such a good job on our first one that I'm holding you responsible for a second child just as beautiful." In this oblique fashion, both men indicated that they knew Maureen was in Dr. Frank's office receiving the sperm that Grant had just produced. They were remarkably calm and cool about the unusual situation they found themselves in.

Almost five years have passed, and the Fogler family is thriving. Grant did not meet his second child, but there is a good possibility that he will sometime in the future. Evan and

106

Maureen are exceedingly comfortable in discussing donor insemination. Evan has no hesitation about telling his children the truth of their conception when they are old enough to understand. He feels virtuous and personally fulfilled by his decision to block his own reproductive capacity. He also seems certain that his children, when they understand his motives, will applaud the decision. There is no question, Evan would tell you, that he is the real father of his children.

COMMENTARY

In the past seven chapters, we focused on donor insemination used by couples when faced with the man's infertility. The special problems of infertility were discussed as they affected the husband, the wife, the donor, and the donor offspring.

In this chapter, fertility and its emotional effects are no longer an issue. Evan was fertile. At least, he was never proven infertile. He assumed that he could impregnate a woman; in fact, he was concerned that he might impregnate a woman who would bear his child. He did not suffer from feelings of inadequacy or from blows to his masculinity. On the contrary, he is a man with a very good sense of self and manhood.

Evan made a choice, based on evaluation and reevaluation over a period of many years. Although he was a young man when he elected to have a vasectomy, his decision was reasoned and mature. For him, the use of donor sperm was free of conflict.

In cases involving genetic disorders, the dynamics are totally different than those involving fertility disorders. This is particularly true when the genetic disorder is known throughout the life of the individual. Evan deplored his diabetic childhood, and he further deplored the idea that another child, especially one of his own, might have to suffer in the same way. It is almost as though he would have lived his childhood twice over were he to produce a diabetic child.

In our experience, couples who choose to adopt because of genetic problems seem to have less difficulty in accepting the

107

need for adoption than do infertile couples. They know that the children they could have borne would have presented greater problems than any they might adopt. For example, a woman who has grown up with a brother, a cousin, and an uncle with muscular dystrophy may not find it difficult to consider adoption. She has witnessed her mother, aunt, and grandmother devoting their lives to caring for helpless, dying boys. She knows that she is a carrier of the disease and could spend the rest of her life in the same manner. The only way for her to avoid that fate is to avoid having her own children.

Of all of the couples we interviewed who had donor offspring, those faced with eugenic problems were, without question, the most comfortable and the most at peace with each other and their children. The relationship between the husband and wife has not been affected by the use of donor insemination. The husband is better able to assume the father role and to set limits than is his infertile counterpart. He does not feel inadequate. He does not feel inferior to the donor. He feels instead that through the donor, he has given those children a gift: a chance for a disease-free life. He is their benefactor, and they are his children.

Although there are no hard figures, it is our experience that in approximately 10 percent of the donor-insemination families, genetic disorders are the reason for the choice. Now that prenatal tests can isolate some birth disorders, more couples bearing potential genetic problems may elect to try to have their own children, terminating those pregnancies that carry the problem genes. As yet, however, most genetic disorders cannot be identified through pregnancy testing.

Evan and Maureen are unique in many ways. They pioneered a new approach to a system that has been closed and secretive for almost a century. They added to our knowledge of the value of openness in donor insemination. They taught us to recognize that such openness could be applied to all participants. We had long championed an open approach in the field of adoption, and we had made the connection of openness to donor insemination before we began our research. How open, however, became more clearly defined for us because of the Evans and Maureens we studied.

Had he known or
dreamed that in
another life he
would start another
family, he certainly
would not have had
a vasectomy.

9 I Had a Vasectomy

"It isn't fair to Arnold. He would have had second thoughts about marrying me if he figured I would get bent all out of shape wanting a baby." Gwen was not sure of what to do. For the last few weeks she had been going back and forth in her mind about this "baby business." In some ways, it was a surprise to her that she was so eager to have a baby. She had tried in vain to push her feelings away, and now she was feeling desperate.

Arnold and Gwen had known each other for seven years and had married four years ago. When they met, Arnold was forty-seven, and Gwen thirty-one. Arnold, a CPA, had been recovering from an acrimonious divorce and feeling bitter toward women. He had three children—two girls, thirteen and sixteen, and a boy, twenty—and a heavy alimony and child-support burden. Gwen, a career woman, had never been married and was intent on becoming the best financial consultant to nonprofit institutions in the Midwest. They met while working together on a funding project for a large public foundation. They were friends long before they became lovers.

When they decided to live together, marriage was a "maybe," because it was frightening to Arnold and unimportant to Gwen. She had little interest (she thought) in a family, and that made Arnold's situation appealing to her. He had all the children he wanted. After the birth of his third child, he had elected to have a vasectomy. He had been almost thirty-five years old, and he wanted to be finished with babies and bottles and night feedings and chicken pox. His wife was against using the pill, and he had been afraid that she would accidentally get pregnant again. Their sex life had not been good of late, and he had hoped that removing the worry of pregnancy would bring back some of the earlier romance.

The vasectomy was not a sudden decision. All through the last pregnancy, Arnold had weighed the pros and cons. Even if something should happen to one of his kids, he could not replace the child, and he wouldn't want to. His wife complained a great deal about raising children and expressed her desire to make something of her life other than stirring chocolate pudding and wiping runny noses. Arnold prided himself on being a feminist supporter. After having three babies, he should take the responsibility for pregnancy off of his wife's shoulders. A vasectomy was an office procedure and carried little medical difficulty or trauma. Their family was complete, and they could raise their children and begin to travel and to enjoy life. It cost so much to raise and educate children these days that three was more than enough. His wife could go back to college, or get a job, or do anything she wanted to once the youngest was in school and she had enough free time.

It was a good plan, and it had worked for almost a decade. Arnold had never regretted his decision to have the vasectomy. While their sex life did improve for a few years, eventually it deteriorated as part of the general collapse of their relationship. They treated each other badly, and the separation and divorce were angry and ugly. Arnold blamed his wife, and she blamed him. They tried to shield the children, and they partially succeeded. As time passed, they learned to cooperate with each other on the children's behalf and to behave in a civil manner.

*   *   *

When Arnold met Gwen, he was beginning to feel like a desirable but dehumanized object on the marketplace. Women were pursuing him; friends were fixing him up with blind dates; colleagues were inviting him over to meet their sisters-in-law. He felt like an adolescent again, but this time around, he knew how to dress and he needn't worry about acne. For almost a year, Arnold had welcomed all of the attention. He dated and bedded women of different shapes, sizes, and personalities. What had initially seemed exciting and validating was becoming boring and meaningless. He wanted to stop having to go through the courtship rituals over and over again. He was ready for monogamy once more.

Gwen was a refreshing change. She was straightforward and honest. Their friendship grew into a deeper closeness and finally into physical intimacy, with underlying trust and commitment. Although there was a sixteen-year age difference between them, Arnold was not worried; Gwen was mature and sensitive, and he felt that they understood each other and wanted the same things out of life.

However, Gwen was young enough to have children, and Arnold was disturbed that she would be giving up that option by choosing a life with him. He had all the children he wanted; he had experienced parenthood with its pleasures and problems. At this time in his life, he was finished with domesticity and suburbia. In Gwen, he had found a life partner with whom he could have a close adult relationship combined with fun, travel, romance, and intellectual companionship. He knew what he wanted, but it worried him that he might be depriving Gwen of experiences that should be available to her. Five or ten years from now, would she resent having married him?

Gwen and Arnold spent long hours talking about the matter. Gwen felt that she had little desire for domesticity. She did not see herself as a woman with overwhelming maternal needs. She had never played with dolls as a child; in all the children's games, she had been the nurse or the teacher, never the mother. She loved her work, and now that she

111

had begun to travel, she wanted to see the world. Raising children was a job too important to leave to others, and yet she did not want to stay home and do it herself. She did not deny that under other circumstances, she might consider having one child: if Arnold had no children; if Arnold were thirty-seven instead of forty-seven; if they were both on the same wavelength. There were none of those ifs.

Gwen convinced Arnold that she was entering into the relationship with open eyes. She loved him and knew that they could be happy together. Arnold wanted to be convinced, and she had agreed that they ought to live together first to see if she would continue to feel as she did. The first few years were idyllic. Gwen assured Arnold that she could live a perfectly contented life without having children. She enjoyed his children and developed a warm relationship with them. Most of their free time, however, was spent without the children, leading an adult existence: traveling, dining out, shopping, and feeling totally free.

Getting married was the next step; their relationship seemed stable and permanent. Arnold had no doubts in his mind; he knew he could not ask for a better life than he had with Gwen. Marriage didn't change their existence except that it deepened their commitment and enhanced their sense of security and trust with one another. They appeared to their friends as an ideal couple who knew how they wanted to live and did so with elan and gusto. Gwen was not defensive about her childlessness. She spoke with candor about her fun as a stepmother and felt fortunate to live in an era when women could choose not to have children without feeling guilty about it. Arnold reveled in his good fortune and praised his wife and their relationship to everyone.

The years passed quickly. With each anniversary, they toasted their marriage and felt that they had miraculously found each other. Gwen felt herself forever young and pretty through Arnold's eyes. They had made a circle of friends whose lives were similar to theirs. Occasionally, when a couple in their friendship circle decided to have a child, the others wondered why. Eventually the new family wandered away from the group, to be replaced by another childless couple. Gwen did not consciously envy those friends who had babies. Occasionally, at a baby shower, she would find herself looking at the tiny sweaters and booties, aware of tears behind her eyes. Occasionally she would hold a friend's baby and smell the talcum powder and feel nostalgic and sentimental. Occasionally she would celebrate her birthday with the overwhelming feeling of time passing too fast.

It wasn't that life stopped being as good. It wasn't that her love for Arnold waned. It wasn't that her career became less important. It was hard for Gwen to pinpoint exactly what it was. Little feelings of discontent began to invade her consciousness. She wanted something, but she couldn't allow herself to know what it was that she yearned for.

At her annual gynecological checkup, the doctor praised her for keeping in such good physical condition. He told her that she had the figure of a twenty-eight-year-old instead of a thirty-eight-year-old. He was not complimentary, however, about her medical condition, feeling that she would probably have an early menopause. He wondered about her mother's age at the onset of menopause. To Gwen, this was an astonishing announcement. The doctor seemed to have forgotten about Arnold's vasectomy and their decision to remain childless. He sat her down in his office to talk with her after the examination was completed.

Forcefully and directly, the doctor advised her that if she wanted a baby, she would have to have it soon. Time was running out. Although at her age she would already be a high-risk pregnancy patient, new knowledge and techniques provided relative safety. If she were carefully monitored, she could have a healthy baby within the next year or two, no later. Gwen started to explain why this was not important to her, but suddenly she found herself tongue-tied. Her heart was pounding, and she felt flushed and uncomfortable. She thanked the doctor and left the office as soon as she could.

The doctor's words kept coming back to her. To her great surprise, tears would begin rolling down her cheeks. Choked up, she sniffled and gulped and tried to control her feelings so that Arnold would not see her behaving in this way. How could she explain what was wrong when she wasn't even sure herself? She started having strange dreams that woke her in a terror. On the bus, walking down the street, standing in the checkout line at the market, she found herself staring at the children and babies, wanting to pick them up.

Once or twice Arnold found her crying silently and he could not get a satisfactory answer from her. Worried, anxious, he remembered that she had been to see the doctor. In his mind, he wrote the worst scenario, one in which she had been told of a terminal illness, which she was keeping a secret from him. He called the doctor and asked him what had happened at her appointment. What was wrong with Gwen? The doctor was quite casual as he assured Arnold that she was physically fine. He went on to recall their conversation about her need to have a baby now if she wanted to have one at all.

For Arnold, the doctor's words were a great relief. He had thought Gwen was dying, and all she was crying about was that she had realized that she wanted to have a baby. He showed up at her office unannounced and took her off to lunch to talk about the secret she was keeping from him. Gwen started crying all over again.

"I promised you that I wouldn't want any children," she said between tears, "and I thought I never would. I don't know why I've changed, but I only know that suddenly it's important to me to have a baby. What should we do? Please forgive me. I know I promised."

Arnold told that her he was not surprised now that he had had time to think about it. "If you remember, I'm the one who never believed that you would be satisfied with not having any children. I'm not happy about starting with babies all over again, but after all, if that's what you really want, that's what counts for me, because I love you." Arnold continued thinking out loud with Gwen. He did not need to remind her that because of his vasectomy he could not father her children. Should they adopt?

Gwen was stunned and elated by Arnold's attitude. When she heard him mention adoption, she found herself spouting information that she didn't know she possessed. Somehow over the years, she had heard and stored facts for this moment. She began to tell him what she thought they could and should do. She had heard of a doctor in the next state who was considered a leading expert on the reversal of vasectomies. What she wanted the most was to be able to have Arnold's baby. First of all, they should ask their doctor for a referral to the expert for his evaluation. Gwen was somewhat timid as she asked Arnold if he would agree to that, and relieved when he quickly acquiesced.

Once Arnold had consented to the idea of a new family, he wanted to get started as quickly as possible. Although Gwen was optimistic about the reversal, Arnold was more realistic. He knew the percentages of failures, but he also knew that if it didn't work, they could arrange for donor insemination. The most important thing to him was to make sure that his beloved Gwen had a baby. He would love the child because it was hers.

In the months after the reversal, while they waited to see if the surgery had been successful, Gwen and Arnold became even closer. Arnold found himself happy to have another opportunity for fatherhood. He had money, leisure, and experience, and he could really enjoy a child this time. Gwen was sad and depressed when they learned that the operation had not been successful, but Arnold took it rather well. He had prepared himself for the disappointment, and now he wanted to move forward into donor insemination immediately. The urgency was to help Gwen have a baby before time ran out. Gwen wondered if Arnold was going along with the idea only to please her; if it wasn't his baby, how would he feel about it, after all?

Arnold could truthfully admit to himself that he wished the child could be his, but since it could not be, he would make the best of the situation. After all, he already had children, and he had had the experience of seeing his own children born. He was a lot better off, he reasoned, than men who had never been able to have children of their own.

Gwen's doctor was very sympathetic and arranged with the sperm bank to provide the donor sperm. It took four months of an insemination series for Gwen to achieve conception. To Arnold, her pregnancy and delivery were memorable experiences. He felt protective, almost fatherly, toward her. Having been through this before, he knew what she needed from him; he may not have been as helpful and sensitive when he was younger.

In the beginning, Arnold felt uneasy about telling his family and close friends of Gwen's pregnancy. It was a little embarrassing to him. Gwen's excitement, however, was contagious, and he had found himself proudly announcing the coming birth. He even told Gwen that he knew that his colleagues were jealous that he, at his age, could become a new father. It was almost as though Arnold shared the experience so empathically with Gwen that he was convinced he had played a major role in the conception. Somewhere in this, the donor insemination had taken on its own special meaning, becoming part of the reversal of Arnold's vasectomy.

Neither Gwen nor Arnold was overly sensitive about sharing with close friends and relatives the story of their attempt to reverse the vasectomy and the subsequent donor insemination. Arnold ruefully admitted that had he known or dreamed that in another life he would start another family, he certainly would never have had a vasectomy. He bragged about the virtues of the donor as described by their doctor, and vowed to live up to the super baby they were producing.

After they became accustomed to impending parenthood, they stopped talking about the donor insemination. Without any specific agreement, they understood tacitly that they wanted to put the information away. This feeling became even stronger after their daughter was born. The baby needed all the protection and security they could provide, which included feeling full membership in the family.

They mentioned the donor father only a few times during the first year of their daughter's life. Their feelings were confused, but not troublesome. The donor insemination was not a secret, and yet it was becoming one. Other people knew about it, but if Gwen and Arnold stopped talking about it, the others would probably forget. They wished their child would never have to know, but if she did find out, they could tell her how much they had wanted her. She was so little and defenseless, and so many years lay ahead before any of this might become an issue. Why worry now?

COMMENTARY

Gwen and Arnold's story is not unusual. The number of vasectomies has increased as a method of birth control since the 1960s. As society focused on the problems of over-population, not only did the number of large families decrease, but it became increasingly acceptable for the male to take responsibility for limiting the family's growth. Until this decade, sterilizing women through tubal ligation involved major surgery, whereas vasectomies were much simpler to perform. They were done on an outpatient basis, with a rapid recovery and little risk. (Today both tubal ligations and vasectomies can be performed on an outpatient basis.) Additionally, with the rise of the feminist movement, more women expected their husbands to assume equal responsibility for birth control.

As vasectomies become more common, vasectomied males face new issues in divorce. Remarriage for such a man has built-in restrictions, particularly remarriage with a younger, childless woman. Having experienced parenting, the man does not see his marriage as necessarily having to include children. In fact, he usually thinks of his second marriage as an opportunity for a different kind of relationship. Instead of family life, oriented around children's needs, he visualizes an adult life, filled with freedom and excitement. Coupled with this, of course, is the continuing responsibility toward the children of the previous marriage.

The childless second wife is expected to accept the husband's children and prior commitments. The contract between the vasectomied male and his new, childless wife implicitly includes her agreement to become a stepmother to his children and to forgo having her own children. Initially, this is not only acceptable to the new wife, but often appealing and rewarding. She has a ready-made family and sees herself in the role of a friend to the growing children. The husband usually perceives this as a permanent and satisfactory arrangement.

There are many reasons for the wife in this kind of family to change her mind about childbearing. However, what we found to be common in these situations was the need the wife ultimately had for a child of her own, one whom she gave birth to within the relationship with her husband. This desire often came as a surprise to her; she had been unaware of such feelings within herself. Because of her biological clock, there was a built-in time limitation. For the husband, not only was his wife's sudden longing for a child breaking the agreement, but it was making him accept a new kind of parenting.

In our research, we found that the women had done an excellent job of convincing their husbands that it was a good idea to have another child. The husband often had to be reassured that he would not be given additional burdens to bear. The wife promised that either she would take on primary responsibility for parenting or she would use support systems, such as nannies and housekeepers, so that the marriage relationship would not suffer.

Once the question of having children was settled, the means had to be resolved. When it was possible for the vasectomy to be reversed, biological parenting was the first option. The percentage of success in reversal surgery is limited. When it failed, or when the man chose not to attempt surgery at all, donor insemination was the second choice. For the vasectomied male, donor insemination did not carry the emotional undercurrents that it did for the infertile male.

In our study, vasectomied males described themselves repeatedly as being sorry that they had given up their procreative abilities and wishing that they had not been so hasty. If they could have changed history, they would have used other forms of birth control and retained their fertility. Given the current technology, they would have had sufficient sperm frozen prior to their vasectomy. However, since this did not apply to our interviewees, they had used donor insemination without great difficulty. All of these vasectomied males had been fertile and had electively ended their fertility. They may have felt that they made a stupid decision, but they did not feel inadequate or powerless.

This does not mean that the vasectomied males were totally comfortable and open about their donor offspring. They were more comfortable and open than were their infertile counterparts. They were less comfortable than were their counterparts with poor genetic histories. They had not felt particularly secretive about the vasectomy when it took place or during the period between their marriages. In almost all of the cases, the couples did not decide on secrecy at the time they decided on donor insemination. The two decisions were separate, and somehow unrelated.

In the case of the infertile male, the secret covers the fact of the infertility and protects the husband. In the vasectomied male, the secret is perceived mainly as a protection for the child. It is usually only a partial secret, known to some, unknown to others. The couple has no guidelines on dealing with the parentage issue for the child. They hope that they will never have to face it but feel that if they do, they will turn to experts for help.

In our study, we learned of some significant differences between the fertile and infertile males. In most of the cases we saw, donor insemination did not adversely affect the vasectomied male's relationship with his wife. In a stable marriage, the balance of power did not shift after the birth of the donor offspring. The father did not feel as detached from the child as his infertile counterpart did.

Although most of the vasectomied men had not expected to raise any more children and were initially reluctant to agree to donor insemination, the results were surprisingly positive. They enjoyed the experience in a different way than with their first parenting. They felt more mature, less stressed, more affluent, and better experienced in dealing with children. This second chance they saw as warm, rich, and rewarding. They spent more time with their children, tried to avoid some of the mistakes they felt they had made previously, and delighted in the relationship. A number of the men were grandfathers as well as new fathers, and they approached this dichotomy with humor and ease. They also saw themselves as retaining youth longer through dealing with a young child.

We interviewed the principals in a number of cases where vasectomied men had divorced the mothers of their donor offspring. Interestingly, divorce cases in our study, whether involving fertile or infertile males, presented similar problems. Secrecy emerged as the main weapon of aggression in these situations, and it could be utilized to hurt the child. Secrecy may be a lesser issue in the vasectomy cases, but finally it must be dealt with and resolved if the child's relationship with his parents is to develop in a healthy way.

10 Lesbian Couples Can Also Have Children

This meeting had been postponed and canceled at least a dozen times. The invitation list had changed again and again. Finally it appeared that we might really meet: a researcher and five lesbian couples, each couple with a child or children. The lesbian couples were somewhat reluctant attendees, but they gained confidence from being in a group with other couples in similar circumstances.

In telephone conversations, when they had begun to back off from coming, we had used soft persuasion by urging them not to disappoint the others who had promised to come. The need for us, as researchers, to learn from them was a point we had stressed repeatedly. In retrospect, the researchers were naive and simplistic, while the women were realistically distrustful, frightened, and strongly self-protective. How much the participants learned from the researchers is unknown. It is, however, clear that we had a great deal to learn from them. In conjoint sessions and group meetings, we continued interviews with lesbian couples who were co-parenting children conceived through donor insemination.

None of the couples had met prior to the meeting. As

they talked, however, they discovered that they had friends and colleagues in common and that they had heard of one another. Obviously, they shared the same sexual preference and had many mutual interests. All of them were intelligent, verbal, and achieving women. They were strong and unconventional in their attitudes and their way of life. They were politically aware and active. They favored donor insemination because it had offered them the opportunity to have children without engaging in sexual relations with men and because it allowed them parental control over the children without fear of harassment or litigation from a biological father. They were interesting women, with interesting backgrounds. As we went around the circle, each couple gave a description of themselves and their lives with their children.

WILMA AND JOANNE

• Wilma and Joanne, in their thirties, are professors of medieval English literature. Wilma teaches at the local Catholic university, and Joanne teaches in the community college system. Wilma is a black woman, beautiful and exotic. She is tall, regal, and dresses in long, flowing garments. Joanne, fair-skinned and British-looking, gives the appearance of having stopped thinking of clothes during her freshman year in a preppie Eastern college. She is still wearing Peter Pan collars under Shetland sweaters, and pleated skirts and penny moccasins.

Joanne gave birth to an interracial boy eight months earlier, whom she is still nursing. Wilma had read about stimulating her breasts to produce milk so that she too would be able to nurse the baby, even though she had not gestated. They had thought that it would be a real symbol of co-mothering, and they were disappointed when it didn't work; Wilma did not produce any milk, even though she had followed the instructions carefully. She had desperately wanted Joanne to have an interracial child, but she had not felt that she had any right to insist upon it, so she had said nothing about it. For Joanne, there never was any doubt. If they were raising a child together, it should be a child reflecting both of them, and that child had to be a combination of white and black. They have lived together as a couple for the past two and a half years, and they feel deeply committed to one another and their child.

They asked a good friend to help them locate the donor and to act as the go-between. For them, that role meant not only finding the right person, getting all of the pertinent information, and asking for medical tests that would ensure the donor's health, but also holding the identification data so that the donor father could be located at any time if necessary. While they know a lot about the donor, they feel that his identity is confidential and not a matter they share with anyone else. There is no question in their minds that their son will be given that birthright information when he is older. A nurse-practitioner friend helped them with the insemination process, which was repeated for several months before pregnancy was achieved.

Wilma and Joanne took turns talking, with one finishing the other's sentence at times. There was a good-natured camaraderie between them, with much warmth and affection. They come from very different backgrounds and cultures, but since their families are estranged from them, they are now trying to bridge cultural differences by building their own cross-cultural environment. They have many friends, both heterosexual and homosexual, and find acceptance in the academic world. Their son will have many good male role models among the friends who have volunteered to be actively involved in his growth and development.

Wilma has no desire to have a baby, but she would be delighted if Joanne wanted to have another child. They have thought about the future, particularly in relation to the child. What if they were to separate? Wilma feels so close to the child that she has no doubt that she would want to maintain a close relationship with him even if she were not living in the home. Joanne believes this and has assured Wilma that she would make it very easy for her to remain in the child's life.

KAREN AND SYLVIE

● Both Karen, thirty-two, and Sylvie, fifty, are Caucasian and Midwestern. They look more like mother and daughter than lovers. Pleasant-looking, they have open, honest manners that are immediately appealing. Neither of them uses much makeup, nor do they seem concerned with outer appearances. They were simply dressed in dark slacks and tailored shirts. Sylvie was a nun for twenty years, leaving the order when she was forty. She met Karen shortly afterward, and they have now lived together for almost seven years. They have two children, a girl of five and a baby less than one month old. Sylvie is employed as a psychiatric nursing supervisor, and Karen is currently taking a semester off from her teaching job in an elementary school.

Sylvie's younger brother was the donor for both children. It took a lot of convincing before he and his wife agreed to the procedure, but Karen and Sylvie feel that it was a good decision. The children carry genes from Sylvie, their aunt, as well as from Karen, their mother. The women come from different religions and different life-styles. Karen's father is a fundamentalist minister who feels that his daughter is hell-bound. Her mother could be more accepting of her daughter, but not while she lives with the father. Karen's siblings have been admonished by the father to disown Karen or they will also be sinners, and hell-bound. Sylvie's family—large, Irish, and boisterous—shrugs it all off and accepts the women and their children. Karen now feels that Sylvie's family is her family, too. They put the brother's name on the birth certificate as father, because that's the truth and because their children will know all about it when they are old enough to understand. Another brother is the godfather of the older child, and a sister is the godmother of the baby.

In some ways, Sylvie's family seems a lot happier about her now that she is openly lesbian than they were when she was a nun. Even though they consider themselves good Catholics, they cannot see giving up the joys in life to retreat to a nunnery. They never understood Sylvie's "vocation" and were delighted and helpful when she decided to leave that pursuit.

Initially, Sylvie's family met and accepted Karen as just a good friend of Sylvie's. Sylvie had always been so quiet and retiring that they were pleased with her new friendship and apparent happiness. Later, as they slowly learned the true nature of the relationship, they accepted it with little outward difficulty. Sylvie's family is close-knit and its members take care of each other. In this context, the women and their children are part of the larger whole. The children have many aunts, uncles, cousins, and grandparents. The family members live close to each other and there is much visiting, mutual assistance, and celebration of birthdays and holidays. Because of this, neither Karen nor Sylvie worries about the children's future.

LOU AND EMMA

● Lou, a twenty-nine-year-old legal secretary, has been living and working with Emma, a thirty-seven-year-old criminal attorney, for the past four years. They are a good-looking pair, slim and casually fashionable in their well-tailored designer jeans, high-heeled boots, and silk shirts. They live in a renovated Victorian mansion that has been converted into a large apartment for their family and two smaller apartments that are rented to friends. Their family consists of Emma's fifteen-year-old daughter from an early marriage, Lou's sixteen-month-old daughter, conceived through donor insemination, a fifty-three-year-old housekeeper, two dogs, three cats, and a large turtle. They are a high-spirited pair who give the impression of feeling on top of the world.

Their good humor was infectious and they had the group laughing as they described the hectic environment of their household. Emma's daughter, Avril, is utterly boy-crazy at the moment and driving them both batty. She is, however, totally comfortable and cool when explaining her family to her boyfriends. Lou's little girl, Sarah, is an indulged, pampered child, with four mothers bidding for her attention. They gave a great deal of thought to the choice of a donor and had a number of offers at their disposal. Finally they chose to use a sperm bank and an anonymous donor because it seemed simpler and less potentially intrusive. They worked with a lesbian obstetrician who was enormously helpful.

Since Lou and Emma's lives are so deeply intertwined, they don't see how they could ever untangle them enough to split up, even if they wanted to. By now, they not only work together and are officers in the same legal corporation, but they own property together and have invested in several restaurants. Seriously, they say, they have a good thing going now and they hope it continues. However, they are sufficiently realistic to know that things do change and that you can never be sure of tomorrow!

ANN AND DARLENE

• Ann and Darlene are two fiery, diminutive Jewish women in their early thirties—one from New York, the other from Idaho—who met in the Pacific Northwest when each was trying to find a nuclear-free environment. They have lived together for five years and have moved several times, attempting to find an ideal community for themselves and their family. Each now has a child, sired by the same donor, so their children are not only being co-mothered, but they are genetically half brothers. Both women are Phi Beta Kappas and come from scholastically achieving families. They seem simultaneously naive and worldly. They run a small but successful consulting firm specializing in grantsmanship and grant writing, and they are savvy about knowing where the foundation dollars are to be found. At the same time, they seem to be wide-eyed and unnerved at the attitudes and behavior of relatives, friends, and acquaintances. Professionally, they are in good control. Personally, they find themselves continually "screwing up" badly.

Ann had her son four years earlier than Darlene did; Darlene was not sure that she had the courage to confront her family with a child as well as her new life-style. Ann has adopted an "I-don't-give-a-damn" attitude with her parents and siblings, who live far away. She sends them pictures, occasional letters, and tries to visit at least once annually.

Her family has decided to "live and let live," according to Ann, and happily, her little boy, Marty, is loved by the whole Idaho clan.

Darlene's experience with her family was quite different in the beginning, but now Teddy, her little boy, has reconciled them. For several years she took Ann and Marty home with her on vacations and holidays, because they were her family. Her father always became embarrassed and uncomfortable when Ann nursed Marty at the dinner table and usually left in the middle of the meal, looking like he "wanted to throw up." When Darlene insisted that Ann's baby was also hers and said that her parents should accept Marty as a grandchild, they told her she was crazy. The relationship was at a stalemate until Darlene faced her parents with her well-advanced pregnancy. Initially extremely upset, her parents had to find a way to accommodate the unconventional and unacceptable relationship into their family, because there was no way that they could deny their first grandchild. They might not accept Marty and Ann; they might not accept Darlene's sexual preference and way of becoming pregnant, but a grandchild is a grandchild without any doubt.

Darlene's maternal grandparents were excluded from the family communication network because they were too old to adjust to new life-styles, although it "almost killed" Darlene's mother to have to keep the first great grandchild a secret. Darlene's parents generously provided the layette and baby furniture, and paced the floor outside the delivery room. They even gave Darlene the down-payment for a house, complete with a yard, in a safe neighborhood.

The man whom Ann and Darlene chose for the donor father was Bryan, a gay computer programmer who lived in their apartment building and had always seemed to be pleasant in a quiet, retiring way. They were looking for a man who would provide them with the necessary genetic material and then recede into the background. They had read an article in a lesbian magazine that explained in detail the method of self-donor insemination, using a turkey baster with which to insert the semen into the vaginal canal. For

127

Ann, there had to be repeated inseminations, but Bryan was willing and patient. He told his widowed mother, who lived in Florida, about the baby, and she was excited and happy. She wrote to the women and sent them hand-knitted sweaters and booties, much to their discomfort. When Ann and Darlene asked Bryan to have his mother back off, he agreed and they were relieved. However, when she was told by Bryan about another baby to be born, there was no longer any holding her back. She wanted a girl this time, she told Ann and Darlene, and she wanted to be able to enjoy sending gifts, receiving pictures, and coming to visit.

Amazingly, the second insemination "took" the very first time. Not only his mother, but Bryan as well, became more direct and less passive with the birth of Darlene's baby. The women had not anticipated such involvement or they would not have recruited Bryan again. Bryan wanted to be a father person to both boys and to help in the financial aspects of raising them. He made a good living and he wanted to pay the tuition to good private schools and to handle the cost of musical lessons, summer camps, orthodontia, and so forth.

Darlene and Ann had to admit that they had helped to create this "monster" and that they did not know what to do about it. It was not that they feared litigation or an attempt to take away their rights because they were lesbians. After all, Bryan was homosexual also. Rather, they were afraid of intrusion and of having to give control, even partial, to Bryan over the future of their sons. They did not want him in the picture at all, unless it became important to the welfare of the boys.

Ann and Darlene have now changed communities in order to put distance between themselves and Bryan and to find a more friendly atmosphere for the family. Slowly they are beginning to recognize their naivete and their need to become more self-protective and street-smart.

Before relocating, they lived in a lower-middle-class working community. Putting Marty into the local public school had seemed to be a good decision, particularly since the school had an adjunct day-care center for working mothers. It never occurred to them to consider the effect their family would have on the community. How stupid they were! Filling out the application, they crossed out "Father's name" and wrote over it "Co-mother" and inserted Darlene's name. One of the teacher's aides was a neighbor of theirs, and she alerted them to the scandal they had caused. They would not have cared if the hostility had been directed toward themselves, but Marty was an innocent child, and it wasn't fair. They were told that other mothers were admonished by the teacher to keep their children away, because Marty's home was an evil place.

They hope that in their new community, housing a larger population of families similar to theirs, they will be able to avoid such problems. All they want to do for the next decade is to settle down, earn a living, raise their children, keep the father away, and lead a happy life.

PAT AND CATHY

● Pat, forty-one, and Cathy, forty-four, were each married, with children and a conventional suburban life, when they met twelve years ago. For over seven years they lived dual lives, pretending to be happy wives and homemakers, except for the brief interludes that they spent together. Neither of them was willing to risk losing her security, and they might have continued the deception, had not Pat's husband discovered the truth. He was enraged and brutal in his condemnation of his wife and her "deceitful, perverted ways." He told Cathy's husband and assorted family members of his discovery and instituted divorce proceedings and a custody battle. Cathy's husband followed suit, and both of the fathers were awarded custody of the children.

For almost five years now, the two women have lived together, continuing to hope that their children will eventually choose to live with them. The children, three boys and one girl ranging in age from fifteen to seven, are now, after years of legal maneuvers, permitted to visit but not to spend the night in their mothers' house.

Both women were deeply depressed during the first year of their forced separation from the children. They had no contact with them and despaired of ever being given any parental rights. Pat, then in her late thirties, decided that they should have a child through donor insemination to help them bear the loss of the other children. Although Cathy was frightened that such action might further prejudice the courts against them, Pat's need was so great that she acquiesced. They consulted the staff at the local women's medical center and were referred to a physician who worked with a sperm bank. Winifred, their little girl born to Pat, is now almost three, and a delight. She is the child they share in their new life together, which makes her very special to them.

Life has not been easy for them during the past several years, but now, finally, they feel a little more secure. Each is employed and earning money with which to support the new family. Their children are beginning to relate positively to them again. With new friends, a new community, and a support network within the lesbian world, they are slowly overcoming the traumas they suffered. They don't trust the heterosexual world and the legal system, and they don't think that they ever will again. They would rather live the rest of their lives in a protected, closed circle among women whom they can depend on not to hurt them.

After the couples had told their stories, the researcher posed four general questions for the group's consideration, turning the meeting back to the participants with each question.

QUESTION 1. There has been a lot of concern expressed about the potential emotional instability of children raised in lesbian households. Many people fear that these children will grow up to be homosexual, promiscuous, or otherwise unconventional. How do you respond to such fears?

DISCUSSION: Emma, the criminal attorney, and Ann, the grant writer, began talking simultaneously and with intense emotion. Then Emma deferred to Ann, who was familiar with studies of lesbian households. Ann was persuasive in pointing out that most lesbians grow up in stable, conventional, heterosexual households. None of the studies to date are clear on the family relationships (or lack thereof) that might be considered contributory to lesbian or gay sexual preference. The old Freudian interpretations are now, according to Ann, open for reevaluation. If lesbians come out of "square, straight" families, perhaps we can look for "square, straight" children to come out of lesbian families. The group responded with good-natured laughter and agreement. Emma, who had waited patiently to break in, took the opportunity.

"I was married," she began, "for ten years after a *Ladies Home Journal* courtship and a *Bride Magazine* wedding. What could be more conventional on the surface? We had all the trimmings—the home right out of *Architectural Digest*, and the family dinners and celebrations straight out of a Norman Rockwell poster. Believe me, it was a cosmetic cover-up. We never told anyone that my husband was a cocaine addict, that our sex life was rotten because he was impotent nine out of ten times, and that I was secretly turned on by women, not by men. We had a baby in order to continue the cover-up; we knew we were living a terrible lie that we didn't know how to get out of.

"Today, in my so-called weird, unconventional, lesbian life, I'm really much more stable, honest, and conventional than I was then. Lou and I are what we are, through and through, without any surface baloney. My daughter knows that I prefer making love to a woman, but she says that she prefers boys, although we have both agreed that she is too young to act on her desires. Lou's and my little one will grow up as normally as any child in any household, if we can help it. If only there were some way we could convince the rest of the world that it doesn't have to be afraid of us."

Wilma summed up the discussion by reminding everyone that today the definition of the family is no longer the same as it was for our grandparents. Most children nowadays, she said, are being raised by single mothers or in blended families, with a number of step and foster and half siblings coming out of second and third marriages. Therefore, why pick on the lesbian families?

QUESTION 2. Some of the donors are anonymous; some of them are known to you or to an intermediary. What are the advantages and disadvantages of these choices? What role do you who know the donor perceive him playing in your child's life? You who have elected to use anonymous donors, do you wish that your child could have access to identifying information? How important is the donor?

DISCUSSION: Sylvie spoke up immediately. "I know that some people think it was creepy for us to use my brother as the father of both of our children. To us, Karen and I truly had both of the children, because my genes were in there even though Karen was the pregnant one. We know our donor's history, and we know his personality, and we would love for our children to inherit his traits. We also can have access to appropriate medical help in the future, if necessary. What Wilma said is really so true. Why is this any stranger than families whose kids have three stepmothers and six half sisters and never know who their father is married to this month?"

Darlene disagreed with Sylvie, although she understood that the specifics of their situations differed. The presence of the father in the family could, she admitted, have value. However, what she and Ann did has only caused problems, and they don't know that they would ever recommend their approach to anyone else. If they had thought it through, they should have known that they were asking for trouble by using the same donor twice and not knowing how either he or his mother felt about children. Bryan, their sons' donor father, seems to think that he should have a say-so in the boys' future, and they don't want him butting into their lives, even if he does have good intentions. The kids are theirs, no one else's. They have recently heard about a donor father who sued and got visiting rights. Should Bryan hear about the case, he may get ideas. If they could do it over again, they would not know the donor or his identity. All they would want would be background and medical information.

Joanne grinned at the other women and bragged that she

132

and Wilma "had their cake and could eat it, too." They knew all about the donor, and they could locate him if he was needed for medical help or to answer their son's questions. They had used a good friend who was smart enough to pick a good donor and to get all the information. They knew him but he did not know them, which was exactly the way they wanted it. They have no worries about his intrusion into their lives.

Pat felt that Joanne might be putting her head in the sand, thinking she was so safe. If anyone knew, it wasn't much of a secret and it could be breached. Pat and Cathy had had such terrible experiences with the law that they had not only wanted an anonymous donor, they had chosen to deal only with the lesbian community. They would not trust a male heterosexual doctor for any procedure, let alone donor insemination. Maybe, Joanne conceded, if they are able to raise their sons to be open and honest individuals, they will trust a few men in the future. Pat said that it would have been even better had the technology permitted her egg to be treated in such a way that sperm would not have been necessary. The others were interested in hearing more about this, but all felt that it was a technique a long way off.

Karen felt sympathy for the women who saw a known donor as a threat to their security, but she expressed greater concern for the child. "What will you tell your child when he wants to know who his father is? A test tube of sperm? After all, there was a person who filled that test tube, and doesn't your child have a right to know who that person was?"

QUESTION 3. How will you tell your child about the donor father? What did you put on the birth certificate? What have you told your family and friends? What will you put on applications for school admission, medical care, and so forth? How much do you know about the donor father?

DISCUSSION: Karen spoke up again, almost continuing where she had left off in the previous question. "We're damn lucky in our situation because we can have our kids meet their father easily and comfortably, and have them know him as they are growing up. Everything about their lives is different, so this might as well be different, too. What we have going for us is that our whole crazy family is comfortable, and so our kids will be, too."

There was no one answer that received general approval by the group or that fit every situation. All of the women acknowledged the difficulty inherent to donor identification. All of them were clear that their children would know that they were donor offspring and would be given whatever information was available. In those areas, there was no secrecy from the beginning. They would stress the fact that their children had two mothers rather than one mother and one father. "Children are resilient," one of the women insisted, and the others picked up the thread by pointing out that many children weathered far more difficult problems than this one. We are making too much of it, they said.

There was no agreement about how to handle birth certificates or applications. Ann and Darlene, having learned a bitter lesson, admonished the group that the outside world should not be educated at the expense of the children. "Lie on school applications and birth certificates. Those bigots out there can hurt our kids, and our kids should be protected." Some of the other women agreed about school applications but insisted that they would not lie on the birth certificate. They had given the child their last name and left the father's name blank.

QUESTION 4. How do you plan to handle problems arising from discrimination, prejudice, harassment, and generally negative attitudes toward your family? Even though you try to live your lives within a protected, accepting environment, how immune can you really be against the outside world's criticism?

DISCUSSION: Although a variety of approaches was offered, it was generally conceded that children raised in lesbian families needed to become strong enough to deal with disapproval from the outside world. The women knew that within their homes and their friendship circles, they could give adequate security to their children. However, there was clearly no way that they could protect the children on the playground, at the Scout meeting, at the neighborhood birthday party, or in the school classroom. They certainly could make sure that their children had good role models to identify with through men friends or relatives. The discussion broadened when the interracial couple and the Jewish couple began to compare prejudice on grounds of race or religion to prejudice on grounds of sexual preference. Prejudice, they all felt, regardless of how it is focused, is lethal, dangerous, and to be fought with ferocity.

COMMENTARY

In professional literature, popular magazines, and books, more has been written by and for lesbian women who plan to have children through donor insemination than for any comparable group. The lesbian community has tried to study and evaluate its experience and to promote practices that will enhance the functioning of its populace in this area.

Underlying much of this writing is the firm belief that each woman is entitled to free choice regarding childbearing and child rearing, as well as an equal opportunity to use available resources toward realizing her choice. Many of the women we interviewed had lived in heterosexual relationships prior to their lesbian identification. Some of them may not have been clearly aware that having children was their only motivation for marriage. Others, aware of their sexual preference, may nevertheless have wanted children so much that they preferred to repress that aspect of themselves. The lesbian couples who participated in our study were very clear, retrospectively, about their emotional conflicts within the marriage relationship. They were happier and more at peace with themselves with lesbian partners, despite the obvious problems that society presented.

As they talked about their families and their approach to parenting, their conversation did not seem very different from that of a traditional nuclear family. They emphasized the need for both parents to share similar attitudes toward discipline and limit-setting, to agree about money, and above all, to have a mutual desire to parent together. Very different in their family structure was the lack of male dominance and chauvinistic approaches to role identification for their children. The lesbian couples whom we interviewed derived strength from their membership within a supportive and trustworthy lesbian community. This was their large extended family, on whom they depended since the outside world was hostile and discriminatory.

Lesbian couples appear to be exceptionally realistic about their situation. They know that they are accused of unnatural acts and attitudes and that they are perceived as being unsuited to providing a healthy moral environment for children. These women are challenging the traditional concepts of family in even stronger ways than the single, non-lesbian woman does. From a religious point of view, the nuclear family, the cornerstone of society, is being attacked and threatened by these lesbian co-mothers.

The couples whom we interviewed may have represented a special group, but we found them to be thoughtful, sensitive, committed, and responsible parents. Some of them were better able to bridge the lesbian and heterosexual worlds than others, but all of them were intent on helping their children to live in both worlds. Our concern about the welfare of the children was that they might develop a nontrusting attitude toward outsiders. This attitude can be found in all oppressed groups, particularly when they are ghettoized, physically or mentally. As society comes to accept lesbian families, this may not pose a great problem.

The donor presents many faces to the lesbian couple. He is at once their liberator, because he offers them the freedom to have children without sexual intercourse and without the potential interference of a heterosexual man. He, in the ultimate anonymous form, offers them total control over the destiny of their child. The donor, if known, can either be a cooperative, interested, important adjunct to the child, or he can be perceived as an intrusive, controlling, interfering person. At the worst, the donor could be a legal threat to the vulnerable lesbian couple.

The donor's sperm, often recruited from within the male homosexual community, is at once a gift of life and the risk of a potentially fatal illness to both mother and child through the presence of AIDS. Before the AIDS epidemic, donors from the gay community were considered by lesbians as highly accessible and sympathetic. Fresh sperm was believed the most desirable because it was easy to use and to obtain at the right time. However, fresh sperm, to be effective, must be inseminated within two hours of ejaculation. To be sure that there is no AIDS or other disease present in the sperm, the fresh specimen must be cultured for forty-eight hours. The present risk in using fresh sperm is obvious, and donor-insemination procedures in the lesbian community have therefore been changed radically. Lesbians are not only turning to sperm banks, but they are establishing their own medical centers and fertility clinics. The casual, informal, self-insemination is no longer considered safe.

Secrecy, when it is practiced in this community, is different than that practiced in the heterosexual community. There is no secrecy about the child being a donor offspring. There is secrecy only about the identity of the donor. Couples such as Wilma and Joanne say that they are very comfortable in making the identity of the donor available to their child when he is old enough or when he needs to know. A question arises regarding their real openness. If Wilma and Joanne worry about the donor interfering with their family, will they really be relaxed about making him available to their child? However, they do have the knowledge, and they can locate him.

For Lou and Emma, who utilized a sperm bank, locating the donor is not possible. Their child will know that she is a donor offspring but will never be able to find her donor father. This is similar to the situation of the donor offspring we interviewed who had learned the truth but were frustrated because it was a dead-end situation. If any group must be aware of the need of available information for the children, it is the group who practices partial openness and then locks the door. We feel that a child growing up with the knowledge of a donor father needs to know that person as part of his identity formation.

From the lesbian couple's point of view, the donor is usually someone whom they wish to avoid or to place in an inactive, powerless, or anonymous position. However, lesbians should be aware that the situation is different from the child's perspective. If we focus on the child's needs, we become cognizant of the fact that the child has half of his genetic makeup from a person, a man who provided the sperm. This man cannot be ignored, discarded, or eliminated from the child's life. He remains a part of the child's identity. In that context, lesbian couples would do well to incorporate this man into their lives to some degree, on behalf of the child.

11 My Clock Is Running Down

As the report of the school budget subcommittee came to an end, Vince Ferguson, president of the Misty Hills Youth Center, looked down at the last item of the agenda. It had been a long Board of Directors meeting and he was eager to adjourn the session. Turning to Susan Hicks-Brown, executive director of the Center, he raised his eyebrows and pointed to the final agenda item: New-Projects Director. She gave him a half smile and mouthed, "You'll see." He could not remember discussing any pending projects with Susan and he wondered what it was all about. Mentally shrugging, he thanked the subcommittee chairman and addressed the board.

"We are at the final item on the agenda for the meeting. Susan added it after our preliminary discussion, so I join you in being totally in the dark about 'new projects.' Whatever Susan has to share with us, I am sure it will be noteworthy and food for thought. Perhaps she has put it last on the agenda so that we can think about it for our next meeting. Before you begin, Susan, I would like to say for myself and for the other members of the board that it continues to be a great pleasure to work with you on behalf of the youth

139

of this community. You have led us into so many new projects, successful and innovative, and certainly in the best interests of the agency, that we trust you will continue to do so for a long time."

Susan Hicks-Brown smiled in response to the board president's complimentary words. She had heard similar words many times during the six years of her tenure at Misty Hills. Without false modesty, she felt that she deserved the board's support because she had worked hard and had developed good programs. From a small residential program for disturbed adolescents, she had built the agency into a multiservice center, offering both in- and outpatient care. Misty Hills now had a diagnostic center, a remedial school, a family therapy program, and a work-training center. Graduate students in the fields of psychology, social work, and education were placed by several local universities for specialized training. The agency served three hundred families annually and enjoyed an enviable reputation in the mental-health community. Susan Hicks-Brown at the age of forty-one was proud of her professional accomplishments.

She enjoyed a good relationship with both her staff and the board. Warm and friendly, she nevertheless maintained a clear distance and separated her professional from her personal life. Although she was open and interested in people, she was a private person and did not volunteer many details of her own experiences. It is surprising how little anyone at Misty Hills really knew of Susan's life. The oldest of three children in a middle-class family with an alcoholic father, Susan had developed a secret inner life early. By the age of ten, she knew that she wanted to go away to college and live in a dormitory. After she left home at seventeen, she returned only for brief holidays. She had always been aware of her intellectual abilities and had used her brains to gain entrance into another world. She had achieved well academically, winning scholarships and awards.

Susan was a pretty girl and had never lacked for dates. She liked boys as friends but did not let herself get too close to them. When a boyfriend began to want more than a casual relationship, Susan found a reason to stop seeing him. She told herself that she was not ready for anything too deep because she had to finish school, or get her graduate degree, or stabilize her career, or find the right person. There were always good reasons, and the years had passed quickly.

Susan consciously tried to keep her personal life separate from her daily work life. When she left the agency at the end of the day, she wanted to see different people, with different interests. She told herself that if she became too chummy with the board members or the professional staff, she would not be able to exercise authority on the job and that the agency would suffer as a result.

Life was rich and fulfilling for Susan, and she rarely thought about marriage or children. Because she had a number of talents and hobbies, she had developed a wide-ranging network of friends and acquaintances. Among her friends there were many families with children of various ages, to whom Susan was the favorite honorary aunt. She was often told that it was a pity she had no children, because she would make a great mother.

It surprised Susan that she became so depressed and maudlin at reaching her fortieth birthday. It was a turning point in her life for which she was ill prepared. What made it most difficult was that she was rarely ill prepared for anything. She prided herself on having foresight and planning ahead, so that she could maintain control over her life. Given more easily to action than to introspection, she felt that she needed to do something constructive before she sank deeper into depression. She knew that she could not sort out her feelings without help.

Susan located a woman psychiatrist whose opinions she had respected when they worked together at a conference. During a series of appointments over several months, Susan and the therapist explored the depression and its onset. What became quite clear early in the treatment was Susan's desire to have a child before it was too late. How strong this desire was and how to achieve it were questions that took a number of months to unravel. When she began to seriously consider donor insemination, her depression lifted almost immediately. Feeling once more in control, Susan started

141

her research. Although she was not asking anyone's permission to have a child as a single parent, she did want to test the reaction of her family and friends. Because she knew that she would need their emotional support during pregnancy and after the child was born, she wanted them to share the decision with her.

It was heartwarming to receive an enthusiastic response from most of her relatives and friends. Of course there were a few negative and shocked expressions, but most people admired her for her courage and offered to help. She did not ask anyone to keep her plans a secret; on the contrary, she decided that it would be better to let her friends and her family network spread the idea, so that she could get a full sense of how she and her child would be accepted in the various worlds she inhabited.

However, she did not discuss the pending donor insemination with the agency: having a baby, she decided, was a purely personal decision. There were consequences that she might have to face at the agency, since the pregnancy was out of the conventional mode. She realized that she was afraid that the Board of Directors could create a furor among its ranks and in the community if given the opportunity to express its opinion before the fact. She laughed to herself as she visualized the committees and subcommittees that the board could form to discuss the various aspects of Susan Hicks-Brown's potential pregnancy and single parenthood. Think of the reports, and discussions of the reports, at meetings! After she made her decision and after she was pregnant, she would tell them. If, on the other hand, she decided against donor insemination, they need never know anything about it.

Susan's friends and relatives were considerate. They shared the information only with other close friends not given to sensationalism or gossip. Such was their esteem for Susan that they saw her desire as deserving their respect and careful thought. Susan asked a number of the adolescents their opinion, and she tried to answer their questions honestly. Some of the kids thought it was a "groovy idea." Others couldn't figure out why she didn't get pregnant in the usual

142

way. Why have this "donor stuff" when there were plenty of men around who could do the job?

To Susan, the reason to use a donor was quite obvious. If she were in love with a man and wanted to create a life out of that love, that would be the best way, of course. But she was not in love with a man, nor did she foresee falling in love with a man in the immediate future. She needed to conceive a child now, if she were going to have one. She no longer had time to wait and see what the future might bring. To simply select a man she had no feelings for and have intercourse with him repeatedly in order to get pregnant and have his child was not good enough for her. She would not want someone chosen in that way to be involved in raising the child with her, nor would she feel it fair to make a man chosen in that way responsible for a child. To buy a healthy male's sperm for anonymous insemination seemed, under the circumstances, the best choice.

There was one offer that she gave serious consideration, because she could sense the man's desperation. His name was Lucas, and she had been involved briefly but passionately with him during graduate school. He was one of the most handsome men she had ever known, and his physical attraction for her was extraordinary. Lucas knew it, just as he knew that he wielded great power over many women because of his appearance and his sensuality. Susan had felt vulnerable and defenseless in the relationship. She felt that he had taken advantage of her, and emotionally used and abused her and then discarded her. True, they had both been young and he may have grown up since those days, but the memory was still painful.

Lucas, since married and divorced twice, was childless, and now terminally ill with advanced testicular cancer. Prior to undergoing radiation with resultant sterility, he had frozen his sperm. When he heard about Susan's plans, he contacted her, offering his sperm, his name in marriage, legitimization for the child, and his estate for the child's future security. He wanted to assure himself of a small piece of immortality through an heir, and Susan could help him achieve that wish. It was a tempting offer in many ways, but she could not accept it. She did not have good feelings about him. Prior to this, his name had evoked anger and mistrust within her. Now pity was added. These were feelings she did not want clouding the issue. If she could not be sure and affirmative about the father, better he be unknown. The money would have been nice, but she was independent enough to know that she could support her child alone. There were more important considerations than money.

Susan had been Dr. Jorgeson's patient for many years, and she felt comfortable consulting him about donor insemination. Dr. Jorgeson, at the age of sixty, had given up delivering babies, but he still practiced gynecology. He was a warm, courtly gentleman who had always treated Susan with regard, and she had enjoyed her contacts with him. Much to her surprise, this appointment was not at all pleasant. He listened silently to her request, but the expression on his face changed from a quizzical half-smile to a tight, almost forbidding grimace. Susan finished quickly, apprehensive at the doctor's negative stance. Dr. Jorgeson was not even subtle in his denunciation of her desire to have a baby through donor insemination. He told her in no uncertain terms that he was against single women being inseminated and that he offered the procedure only to married women whose husbands were sterile. Children, he continued, should be born into families with fathers and mothers who were married, not to single women who had no husband.

Susan was stunned by Dr. Jorgeson's behavior. She felt attacked and denounced by a professional whom she had always held in high regard. She drove home silently weeping and wondering if she had any right to have a baby. It was a devastating experience, and she was depressed and withdrawn for days afterward. She did not share the trauma with anyone until after her appointment with her therapist; the wound was too fresh and raw. The therapy session helped her to put Dr. Jorgeson's opinion into a clearer perspective and to invalidate his words as a personal indictment of herself. She was able to view him as an individual from an older generation, with a point of view that limited his ability to understand her. She felt that her therapist shared her feelings when she gave Susan suggestions toward seeking other avenues for donor insemination.

Susan did some discreet research and located a fertility clinic whose codirector, a single woman, had helped other single women achieve pregnancies through donor insemination. This experience was positive. Susan felt immediate empathy from the physician and set up appointments to complete the necessary medical tests. She gave a great deal of thought to the kind of donor she would like to have as father of her child. She was delighted that the clinic used medical-school students as donors, because she wanted a person of good intelligence. The clinic personnel were encouraging and reassuring, and she trusted them. She was on her way to having a baby!

By the evening of the Board of Directors meeting, Susan had known of her pregnancy for almost two months. Initially apprehensive that she would miscarry, or be told that it was all a mistake and she wasn't really pregnant, Susan now felt assured. She was one of the lucky ones; she had conceived a child after only three months of insemination. She had been wary of telling anyone that she was pregnant until now, because it would be dreadful to have to take the good news back if she miscarried. Now she was ready to announce it to the world and officially become a happy mother-to-be. For the past week, she had given much thought to the way that she would explain the pregnancy to the board members. Her news had to be carefully told so that it would likely be accepted by even the most conservative members. She wanted to continue working until the birth, take two months off, and then return to full-time responsibility, with a competent live-in housekeeper to look after the baby during the day.

Now, with the board members looking at her expectantly, Susan leaned forward and began to talk. There was a new tone in her voice, and her eyes seemed exceptionally large

145

and luminous. This was a different person than they had known for the past six years. She took them step by step through the realization of her loneliness, her maternal desires, and her decision to seek donor insemination. She shared her family's support with them, and the plans she had that would permit her to continue her work as the Center's director. She asked for their understanding and acceptance. Finally, she told them she hoped that she could use her pregnancy to give the children at the Center a better understanding of the childbearing process as well as a knowledge of the use of donor insemination.

Susan, who had always seemed independent, self-reliant and correct in her relationship with the board members, suddenly found herself emotional and vulnerable, asking them to accept her and to support her. There was silence after she finished speaking. Finally, Vince leaned over and gave her a tender hug. He was followed by the other members of the board, all of whom gathered around her. The silence was broken and there was a great deal of excited chatter and laughter.

In the months that followed, Susan became a symbol to many people. She was treated with deference and respect, and she felt herself very special and very loved. Her growing baby was the subject of much discussion and interest. The boys and girls involved in the Misty Hills Center programs went through every step of the pregnancy with her and became experts on conception, gestation, and birth. The staff related to their director with new warmth; she appeared more receptive to them, and more emotionally open. They gave her advice and tried to prevent her from working too hard. The board members, although not much older than Susan, felt parental toward her and wanted to include her and her child in their family activities. To her friends and family, she was "the one who could pull it off, if anyone could!"

To herself, Susan was an ever-surprising kettle of smoldering feelings and desires. She bought a beautiful leather-bound journal to keep for her child. In it she tried to record the meaning of the pregnancy to her so that one day a grown young person might feel good about having been wanted in such a special way. Susan hoped that this would help to make up for the absence of a father. There were many men willing to be that male figure in the child's life, but that was not the same as a father, and Susan knew the difference. She had to decide what to do about a father's name on the birth certificate. In the end, she, who abhorred deceit, decided to be deceitful and make up a name to fill that space. The child would know the truth, she told herself, but strangers in offices, asking for verification, would have no need to make judgments on an empty space. She could have known the sex of the child after the amniocentesis, but she elected to be surprised. She wanted all the thrills and all the surprises, because she knew that this would be her one and only baby.

For Susan, all of the long-locked doors of feeling had been opened and she didn't think that she could ever close them again. Maybe now she could consider herself open to loving not just a baby, but another person. Maybe she could give herself and her child the gift of a husband and father, a gift that would make them a complete family one day. It was no longer difficult to imagine herself trusting and loving another human being. The donor had not only given her the gift of life through the birth of a child, but the gift of a different and new life for herself as a whole person.

COMMENTARY

Pregnancy, childbirth, and child rearing continue to be perceived by society as the sole prerogative of the married couple. This despite the fact that many children today live in single-parent or blended families and cannot claim to grow up in the home of their birth mother and birth father. The traditional family is becoming the exception.

A woman without a man is, unfortunately, still considered to be incomplete. However, if she is divorced and raising a child or children as a single parent, she is part of a large statistical group, about which much is written; her problems are well-documented. If she is an object of compassion, it is not because she is single, but because she has to fill so many roles: mother, father, and—usually—breadwinner.

Single, unmarried, childless women in our society, however, *are* objects of compassion. Most of these women do not face their limited childbearing years until it is almost too late. Only then, looking at the reality of never giving birth to a child, do they realize how much they want to have this experience. For most of them, donor insemination is not an acceptable option. It requires too much risk-taking. They need to have high self-esteem and courage in order to fight society's traditional mores.

The women whom we interviewed were cut from a special bolt of cloth. They were primarily accomplished career women who had achieved executive or managerial status, with relatively high monetary rewards. They had attained their goals in a male-dominated world through sheer determination and effort, and they were proud of it. They had no doubt that they could take care of themselves. They also felt that alone they could take care of a child, or children, and provide all the necessaries and luxuries. They were not shrinking violets, and they led busy, independent, and productive lives. Nevertheless, they had discovered, as they moved into the second half of their thirties, that something was missing. By the time they had identified their desire, they had found themselves desperate, with little time to waste.

One single, childless woman, a pediatrician in her thirty-ninth year, was asked by the chief of staff in her hospital to consider taking on an additional specialty, because she was so capable. Her reply, which surprised even herself, was, "Right now I'm not planning to hang any more certificates on my wall. The next thing I hang on my wall will be a finger painting made by my own child."

Since adoption is no longer a viable option, with so few healthy, Caucasian babies available and with single women in competition with couples for these children, ever-greater numbers of single women are turning to other options. Marriage is one, but often it is out of their emotional reach. Choosing a man to father a child is difficult and presents other problems that they would rather not have to face. Donor insemination is, for the single woman who would like to have the experience of bearing a child, the simplest solution.

It was interesting for us to discover that the single woman who used donor insemination did not see herself as an "unmarried mother" in the old definition of the term. "Unmarried mother" connotes an unfortunate person who finds herself with an unplanned problem pregnancy, achieved through sexual involvement, usually with a man who has deserted her or has refused to accept responsibility. In contrast, the single parent with a donor offspring presents a picture of a woman who planned her pregnancy and achieved it without sexual intercourse with a man. This woman often inspires great admiration among her colleagues and relatives. Her parents, long despairing of ever having grandchildren, are usually delighted. Adjectives such as "strong," "brave," and "pioneer" are frequently applied to the single mother of a donor offspring.

For that mother and child, the aspect of secrecy is unnecessary. As a matter of fact, it is to their advantage to tell the truth because otherwise the woman will be accused of having had a "child out of wedlock" and of being an "unmarried mother." A number of the women we interviewed kept diaries of the process to share with their child later, because they saw the period as a romantic, emotion-laden time in their life. They ruled out deception, because they felt that the truth was less problematical and more constructive. They were proud of what they were doing. When asked, they did agree that, all things considered, they would rather have fallen in love, married, and had a child out of such a relationship. Short of that, donor insemination was the best solution.

Once embarked upon a course of single parenthood through donor insemination, these women were open and eager for information and advice on the best parenting methods to use with their children. They often reestablished close family ties in order to give their child an extended network of relatives, and they relied upon married siblings and friends to act as important role models. Because they had enjoyed a successful relationship with co-workers, staff, and colleagues, they had no problems in using their environment to the best advantage for themselves and their child.

Most of these single parents had elected to use an anonymous donor because it seemed to be the least complicated for themselves and the child. Without a known donor, the mother retained all legal and custody rights to the child. A known donor, no matter how cooperative initially, might decide at a later date to become involved. If he could prove biological parentage through blood tests, he could ask for joint custody and parental rights. Despite this desire for anonymous donors, the single women seemed to be more concerned with who the donor was than were their lesbian-couple counterparts. They wanted assurance of a healthy, nice-looking, intelligent donor, one whose genes, coupled with theirs, would ensure the birth of a superior child.

They were not concerned with how their child would feel about the anonymity. It was a factor far removed from consideration. However, when offered the suggestion that a child might someday want to find that donor and that such information should be available, they were open to the idea.

At the time of the donor insemination, most of these women had put away thoughts of marriage. A number of them described themselves as emotionally constricted prior to the birth of their child. They perceived themselves as having been totally immersed in career and promotions, and emotionally unavailable to anyone. Loving and caring for a baby was a surprisingly rich experience for most of them, and they felt themselves become more easily in touch with their feelings and more readily open to sharing themselves with others. One woman described herself as suddenly being approached by many men, some of whom saw her as a highly sensuous person, others who wanted children and saw her as the kind of person to whom they could easily relate.

Other women in our study maintained a consistent attitude toward independent single parenthood, feeling no desire to include a father or husband. They felt that they had the opportunity to give clearer messages and directions to the child if there were no one else sharing the upbringing; the absence of a male head of the household precluded any struggle for dominance between the parents. These women wanted to raise their children in their own special way. They did not find themselves suddenly left in a single-parent situation, trying to manage. They had chosen and planned their course carefully.

Studies of single-parent households have not included this group. It would be interesting to compare the various single-mother groups. If it were to be shown that these donor-inseminated single mothers are in fact rearing their children as well as or better than is the traditional nuclear family, it could have significant implications for our understanding of parent-child relationships.

The use of donor insemination is increasing, and it will continue to do so as an option for the single woman; it appears to be utilized fairly openly and aboveboard. The single woman is available to teach us new approaches and to help us redefine our directions on behalf of the child. The knowledge we gain from these single-parent families, we can apply to all of the donor offspring and their parents.

We cannot emphasize
too strongly our deep
conviction that every
donor offspring needs
to know and feel the
donor father as a
human being who
wanted to provide
the sperm that
brought the child
into existence.

12 Ending Secrecy and Anonymity... How and When to Tell

We firmly believe that the practices of secrecy and anonymity must end and be replaced with open identification of the donor father and open knowledge of origins for the donor offspring. The donor father is a real person, not a teaspoonful of sperm. The donor offspring is a genetic product of two parents, with the right to know the truth. The century-old practices of secrecy and anonymity have bred a complex set of problems within the fabric of the DI family. We are convinced that in all DI families, the need to maintain secrecy and anonymity has had an adverse effect upon all of the members.

In the previous chapters, we have attempted to describe the experiences, attitudes, and problems of people involved in donor insemination. Even under the most optimum of circumstances and in the closest of families, the presence of secrecy creates dilemmas. The parents in a DI family live with lies and deceptions, which continually need to be reinforced with more lies and deceptions. Friends and relatives, particularily those of the infertile husband, looking for inherited characteristics in the donor offspring, add further burdens and pressures. Consequently, the nongenetic fath-

152

er's extended family unwittingly often becomes a source of irritation and anxiety to the parents.

Whenever a family lives with a secret, the fear of revelation of that secret is a specter that haunts those holding the information, ultimately straining their relationship. Almost all of the donor offspring whom we interviewed had learned the truth of their origins in a punitive manner, when their parents' relationship began to disintegrate.

In our interviews with the parents of donor offspring, we inquired extensively about their approach to secrets in other parts of their lives. They were candid in describing discomfort and uneasiness with secrets in general. It is interesting that they were almost unanimous in identifying themselves as people who did not lie well, who were impelled to be honest in their relationships, and who basically abhorred deception. However, where the husband's sterility and the use of donor sperm were concerned, they had been indoctrinated and instructed by medical personnel never to divulge the truth to anyone. This fear of ever telling the truth deprived some families of the opportunity to seek adequate help for their problems. Even in so-called confidential environments, they tended either to lie or to in some way avoid revealing the truth about the donor insemination.

The question might be raised, "If a person never knows about having been conceived through donor insemination, how would he be harmed?" That person is harmed in many subtle ways. The parents' conspiracy of silence affects their relationship, which in turn has an impact upon the child. The parental roles shift, and the mother may assume greater authority over the offspring because she is the sole genetic parent. As a result, the nongenetic father may feel less able to parent and to set limits, causing the donor offspring to be deprived of full parenting by his legal father. The donor offspring may internalize the anxiety of his parents and feel somehow responsible for it, and unworthy. From a moral or ethical perspective, each individual should be entitled to know the truth of his conception and his genetic heritage. Essentially, donor offspring are a deprived group who are denied access to information available to the rest of the population.

It is easier to formulate theories and ideal solutions than it is to outline concrete methods of giving complicated information. However, it is important to address these issues, to deal with the problems realistically, and to find adequate solutions. How and when do you tell donor offspring the truth?

Adoption has taught us a great deal about the need for openness and honesty in family relationships. There are similarities between DI and adoption. In each kind of family, the infertile parent must first explore and then accept the loss of being able to produce offspring. To grieve for the inability to create life and to mourn for the child, or children, that will never carry one's genes is necessary. Donor insemination cannot cover up the handicap; it is a viable solution only after acceptance of the handicap is achieved. If the grief is not successfully resolved, it is difficult for the legal father to understand the donor father's role in the child's life.

Adoption and DI have been shrouded in secrecy for many decades. The secrecy has been lifted from adoption, but many adoptive parents still deny the importance of the birth parents' role in the adoptee's life and self-concept. DI is still a secret institution, where the donor father is totally denied in all aspects. Once DI is no longer secret, once the donor is no longer anonymous, the significance of the genetic origin will take its rightful place in the donor offspring's life.

There are also differences in the two institutions that make the imparting of information dissimilar. Adoption is a concept that young children can usually understand. In its simplest form, it can be shared with the child at a relatively early stage of development, usually between five and seven years of age. Donor insemination, on the other hand, is more highly technical and needs to be explained at an appropriate time; it is closely allied to the early understanding of sexual reproduction and intercourse. Donor insemination as a concept is outside the comprehension of any child younger than nine or ten years of age. For some chil-

154

dren, the ability to understand it will be closer to adolescence. For others, disclosure may be more appropriate at the time of young adulthood.

Children's sophistication and capacity for conceptualization vary greatly from family to family and from culture to culture. There is no single rule about the age of disclosure; telling must be geared to the individual child and his family. Although it is possible that there are very young children who could understand reproduction, it is better to err on the later than on the earlier age for telling. If the parent is comfortable in the disclosure of a donor father, a positive feeling about the information will remain, even if the facts are not completely comprehensible to the child. All children need to feel that they are normal and that they are accepted within their families, and this includes donor offspring.

Although donor offspring will not be told of their conception and genetic makeup until at least a decade after their birth, growing up in a climate of openness contributes to healthy familial attitudes and relationships. If the parents no longer live with sealed lips and the outlook of a lifetime of secrecy, they are better able to proceed with the telling of the truth at an appropriate time. In this way, they provide the child with a sound emotional climate from the outset.

We feel that a primary objective is to take the concept of insemination out of the laboratory and to impart the necessary human quality to the giver of the sperm. Therefore we must start with the donor and his role. No more anonymous donors or mixed sperm for insemination means that we eliminate the reservoir of anonymous and mixed sperm in sperm banks. All sperm must be received from known volunteers who agree to share total identifying social and medical information. The donor must agree to be available on a lifetime basis as the genetic parent. This implies updating information, permitting contact with (or on behalf of) the child, and accepting responsibility as an important genetic link for the child.

There are two basic types of DI families to consider in relation to the how-and-when-to-tell question: 1) the nu-

clear family, with a father and mother initially living together, and 2) the families of the single woman and the
lesbian couple. In the nuclear family, the child is born within
the marriage and nurtured by two parents. He assumes himself to be their child and moves through the early stages of
development asking the appropriate questions, which require the answers that any nondonor offspring would receive. The difference arises when the donor offspring becomes
old enough to learn about reproduction, conception, and
sexual relationships that result in pregnancy and childbirth.
Most children who are comfortable in talking with their
parents about special information tend to personalize the
facts and relate them to themselves and their families. It is
not unusual for a preadolescent child to ask parents if the
father's sperm fertilized the mother's egg to produce him
in the way he learned about it in his health class.

Unfortunately, the child often does not give his parents
ample opportunity to prepare answers. These kinds of questions are sometimes posed at awkward times. We are not
suggesting that the parents must explain this personal
and private family information immediately. However,
we are advocating that parents be prepared for the inevita-
ble questions and set aside time for quiet and comfortable
discussion.

The question is a sexual one for the child, and he wants
validation from his parents that he is their child. The donor
offspring needs to be reassured at the time he is introduced
to the concept of reproduction that he has a donor father
somewhere in the picture. We feel that it is appropriate for
the father to let his child know that he was and is sad that
he could not be the child's genetic father. He understands
that the child may also be very sad to learn that his father
is not his genetic father and that he has a donor father. Both
father and child can then share in feelings of loss. There is
no way to avoid pain or discomfort in this revelation. It is
not only appropriate for father and child to confront the
issue together, but also proper that the father aid the child
in the process of understanding, accepting, and healing.

Parents often feel that their role is to protect their child from pain and suffering. We believe that this is unrealistic, and unhealthy for the child. The truth may be initially painful, but dealing with painful situations is an inherent part of life. It should be emphasized that most of the time, parents who are afraid of "upsetting" their children with the "truth" are actually more afraid of upsetting themselves by reawakening old unresolved feelings.

For many children, the initial explanation of DI will need to be as simple and straightforward as possible, because the child will be able to absorb only the broad outlines of what he is told. The three most important elements in the initial revelation are the father's fertility problem, the existence of a person, a donor father, who provided the sperm, and the reassurance of being loved. We cannot emphasize too strongly our deep conviction that every donor offspring needs to know and to feel that donor father as a human being who wanted to provide the sperm that brought the child into existence. Presenting the donor father as the real person he really is provides the child with the grounding necessary to allow him the feeling that he is like everyone else. Donor offspring are normal people, not freaks; they have been conceived in the way that all human life is conceived.

A wise procedure for parents to follow is to first provide basic information and then to elicit questions. Parents should not rush to tell all, but instead, lean back and listen. Listening opens the door to understanding what it is that the child really wants to know and how much information he can handle. Some children may be overwhelmed more easily than others and may need time in which to integrate the information before asking further questions. Parents, recognizing this, can be helpful by leaving the matter open for future discussion; the freedom to bring up the subject of DI later is of great importance.

As the donor offspring grows up, his awareness and understanding of the insemination process increase. Each person is unique, and there is no formula for how and when the child's interest will wax or wane. Being a donor offspring is only one facet of life. The subject may assume more importance at certain times than at others. For example,

157

although the existence of the donor father is a known fact, identifying information may not be necessary until the offspring is older and ready to deal with it. Some children may be intensely curious to know their donor father's name immediately; others may wait until they want to use the information for meeting the person.

What the parents know about the donor father is information that belongs to the donor offspring, although it may be many years before all of it is passed on. Unfortunately, most of the donor offspring of today have anonymous donor fathers and their parents have little information. It is also unfortunate that they cannot get further information since most of the records were routinely destroyed in the past. While telling the child of his origins with only scant information may be difficult for the parents, it is not impossible if approached with the following in mind. Parents must admit to the child that it is sad that they are lacking in information. It is important to convey to the child that they know he would like to have more and that they wish they had it to give. However, what they do know can be shared in a way that, within reason, fleshes out the donor and gives him human qualities and characteristics with which the child can form a degree of identification. Recognizing some of the unique qualities of the child that in all likelihood were inherited from the donor may provide additional feelings of identity. All of this helps the child to feel more comfortable and positive about his donor father and, as a result, about himself.

It is less difficult to set up guidelines and criteria for future openness than it is to address the situation of the tens of thousands of donor offspring who have grown up under anonymity and secrecy. DI parents who can now accept openness are being faced with the need to explain why they did not tell the truth earlier. In its simplest form, the answer is that donor families followed their physicians' advice. Their discomfort with their secrets, and their recent recognition of the donor offspring's inherent rights, foster their decision to share the truth with their DO.

To the nuclear family with an infertile husband, the donor

father was never perceived as other than a donor of sperm who enabled the couple to become parents. He does not have a role in nurturing or parenting; his importance lies in the genetic and historical connection he offers the child. To complete that role, he should be available to his offspring if and when necessary.

When secrecy and anonymity are lifted from the DI family, thought must be given to the question of sharing the information with relatives, friends, neighbors, and schools. It is difficult to make generalities in this area, because families vary in the degree of sharing with which they are comfortable. Some families, nuclear or extended, are very open in all areas, while others have their own rules of privacy, even among close kin. Generally, we believe that it is not necessary to share DI with neighbors, acquaintances, schools, or non-close friends. We would compare DI information with other rather private and intimate facts that belong within the family. On the other hand, we believe that for the parents, to lift the secrecy and to feel comfortable means sharing the truth with grandparents and other close family members. It is important that the parents feel at ease about the material they disclose, because their acceptance of it will facilitate family acceptance. Parents have a responsibility to educate their relatives to a new awareness and understanding of the concept of DI.

There is a fine balance between openness on the part of the parents and freedom to advertise information on the part of the preadolescent child. There is no satisfactory answer, but it is hoped that the sensitivity of the parents toward the needs of the child will help bridge the gap so that the child will know that the information is selectively shared with close friends and relatives. It is a situation not too different from that of the child who learns about reproduction at home and then tells other children about it, some of whose parents are not as openminded. Fortunately, as the child matures, this problem tends to resolve itself.

The second group for whom "how and when to tell" is a major consideration is that of the single woman and the lesbian couple. The main difference here is that in this group, it is not a secret at all. For single women and lesbian couples, the decision to use donor insemination is known to their friends, and often to their employers and colleagues. Also, the donor is often a known person, recruited either by an intermediary or by the mother herself. For our purposes, in discussing "telling," the third difference is in the absence of a father from the home. Because the donor is not usually perceived as a major parenting resource but only as an enabler, he is not generally available to the child. In addition, the unmarried woman utilizing DI is not often eager to give the donor father very much power.

We believe that the same principles regarding the donor father apply to all groups with donor offspring. Every donor offspring, whether raised in a mother-and-father home, a mother-only home, or a mother-and-female-partner home, has an innate right to have a father who is a person. Children raised in fatherless homes generally become curious about their lack when they come in contact with children who have two parents of different sexes. The child who asks, "Where is my daddy?" should receive information about that "daddy." We interviewed many single women and lesbian couples who told us that they answered that question (all of them said it arose by the time the child was three or four years of age) by saying something like, "You don't have a daddy, only a mommy," or, "You have two mommies instead of one mommy and one daddy."

We firmly believe that those replies are not in the best interest of the child. The child does have a father, and he should not be deprived of that person, or of that part of his own identity. It is not important whether the mother wants the father in her life or not. It is important that in some positive way, the child can have a father (like everyone else) in his life. Even if the father never visits or becomes known to the child, his existence and being and personhood should be known and acknowledged.

We know that many people in the lesbian community are deeply involved in studying and writing about this subject. They feel that their problems are unique and need hitherto uncharted approaches and solutions. While this is undoubtedly true, it is also true that many human emotional needs are universal. We hope that our point of view will be considered as they continue to study these problems.

We believe that the difference between the nuclear-family group and the single-mother and lesbian-couple group in "telling" is only in the early stages of the child's development. It becomes an issue sooner in situations where there is no father in the picture. The groups merge at a later stage in the child's maturation. Single mothers and lesbian couples need to introduce the concept of donor insemination when their child learns about reproduction. This knowledge enables the child to more fully understand the role of the donor father in his or her mother's life.

We are convinced that no matter how difficult it may be to change ingrained ideas about donor insemination, ending secrecy and anonymity are in the best interests of the parties involved.

The definition
and meaning
of conception,
gestation, pregnancy,
and parenthood
are changing.

13 Looking Ahead: The World of High-tech Baby Making

The world of high-tech baby making is relatively young. It is in a state of rapid change and development, out of which studies and research projects will undoubtedly be forthcoming. Although our book is focused on donor-insemination families, we felt that it was necessary to address some of the issues that all noncoital reproduction methods have in common.

Throughout the twentieth century, the practice of DI has continued, involving ever-greater numbers of individuals. Because it has been shrouded in secrecy, it has been virtually impossible to evaluate the practice. Consequently, DI, which deeply affects many people, has never been given the opportunity to develop and to meet the genuine needs of the individuals whom it has served. We hope that a similar secrecy, anonymity, and deception will not become institutionalized in the practice of high-tech baby making.

There is great excitement in the media with each new scientific advance that enters the field of conception and gestation. With each new discovery or technique, childless individuals and couples are given renewed hope for achieving parenthood. Our studies of adoption and donor insem-

162

ination have added to our understanding of the desperation inherent to the quest for a child. Individuals will go to almost any lengths and take almost any risks to have a baby. The need for immediate gratification overrides concern for the future. Lifelong implications are ignored. What begins as a desire to start a family becomes an almost irrational obsession.

Unfortunately, the media often present an unreal picture and offer false hope to the infertile person. Much of the experimentation reported is impractical and not available to the general public. Nevertheless, it must be recognized that the definition and meaning of conception, gestation, pregnancy, and parenthood are changing; new methods and their implications are raising a myriad of questions that will require thoughtful, creative answers.

Medical science has developed new techniques for saving very premature babies. The survival rate of newborns at an ever-earlier stage of fetal development is increasing. Simultaneously, fertility experts have found ways of prolonging the life of the fertilized ovum in the laboratory, outside of the human womb. Thus the time span between the viable fertile ovum and the viable human fetus is being shortened, giving rise to the not-too-distant possibility of conceiving and gestating a child in an artificial womb. This scientific engineering challenges our traditionally and universally accepted concept that children grow in and are born from a woman's body.

And there are even more-startling experiments that threaten the fabric of our society as we know it. It is thought possible that males may be enabled to carry and give birth to children; to create a womb in a man's abdominal cavity and implant a fertilized ovum is a technical possibility. In Greek mythology, we have the example of Zeus, the god who gave birth to Athena, born from his head after he swallowed the Titaness, Metis.

Another theoretical concept would make it possible for women to clone themselves and give birth without fertilizing their egg with male sperm. However remote these methods are, they deserve mention, if only to point out how far afield our technology is moving. Unfortunately, there is no consideration being given to the emotional and human implications of these techniques; the focus is solely on medical miracles.

The medical miracle is concentrated on fulfilling the needs of the infertile individual or couple; it allows no room for consideration of the lifelong effect upon the child. Medical science tends to see "progress" in an isolated manner, with little or no awareness of the confusion and the potential disasters that might ensue. Because science shows us that a new direction is possible, it does not mean that this direction should be taken.

It should be noted that despite the wide publicity given to alternative conceptions, the numbers of people involved are still relatively small. The numbers involved in donor insemination, however, are large, and they will continue to grow at a greater rate than that of other methods. DI is the least-expensive procedure to administer, has the same rate of success in conception as that of normal sexual intercourse, and is simple to perform, requiring no special equipment. Throughout its century-old history, DI has proven to be relatively safe and uncomplicated from a medical point of view. From a psychological point of view, this same simplicity has lent itself to institutionalizing deception, secrecy, and anonymity.

Our concern lies in the rapidity with which new technologies are being developed without adequate consideration of their emotional implications. There is a close connection in the emotional effects experienced by all of the parties involved in DI, adoption, and high-tech baby making. Universal human needs for genealogical and historical connections are the same for people everywhere, no matter how they were conceived or gestated. The understanding of who we are, where we came from, and whom we connect with in our past must not be sacrificed in the name of the new era of scientific bioengineering.

High-tech baby making threatens to become "big business," with huge marketing and distribution potential and billions in profits worldwide. The business community uses strenuous techniques to merchandise hamburgers, nuts and bolts, and new perfumes, and soon new ways to make babies may well fall into the category of "merchandising." The goal of any business is to generate a good return on its investment. To ensure profitability, a high-tech baby-making industry must utilize marketing methods and promotional efforts to convince the public of excellence and desirability. The making of large profits calls for high volume, standardization, and development of chains, or franchises. A similar push for volume in the production of babies will only increase the complex legal, ethical, social, and moral questions already inherent to new reproductive methodologies.

Whether we are discussing in vitro fertilization, embryo transfer, surrogate motherhood, or donor insemination, we must keep in mind the universal human needs of the people involved and the necessity to preserve those needs. It should be noted that the more complex the method of conception, gestation, and birth, the more complex the psychological implications and emotional reverberations. We believe that being open and honest, and sharing the facts with the offspring, are universally necessary. The true facts of origins become more difficult for the child to understand and accept in high-tech baby making. For example, when an individual comes into being as a result of a mixture of egg and sperm donors, in vitro fertilization, embryo implantation, and surrogate motherhood, his lineage is obviously confusing. It becomes even more confusing when that same individual has to undergo legal adoption to finally achieve his identity. Integration of the facts and achievement of acceptance and self-worth can come about only with the sensitive help of mature, thoughtful parents. The age at which information is shared depends upon the complexity of the information.

Just as in DI and adoption, the parents involved in high-tech pregnancies will have to come to terms with their own infertility before they embark upon parenthood. Just as in DI and adoption, the donor parent, or parents, must be known and available to the offspring. Just as in DI and adoption, the offspring must be recognized as having another genetic parent, or parents, who are important to him.

We are on the threshold of a wholly new era of high-tech baby making that contains unknowns that we cannot even predict; in addition to the genetic and medical heredity passed to offspring in DI and adoption, we can now add gestational heredity as a potentially important aspect. We do not yet have a clear understanding of the gestating womb, especially when the woman carrying the fetus is not the genetic mother.

The flow of medical information must continue throughout the life of the individuals involved. Indeed, high-tech baby making is a lifelong process that does not end with the creation of the child. Although the method of creation is different than that of normal conception, gestation, and birth, the child born of high-tech baby-making technology is no different than any other human being. He will experience the same stages of growth and development as does everyone else.

Children brought into the world through these new scientific advances must be provided with the the most highly sensitive professional thinking at our disposal. These individuals may be unique and special, but they are also part of the human family, which, in the final analysis, is the most important consideration of all.

14
Recommendations

This chapter is a summary of recommendations based upon the totality of our material. These recommendations have been developed through the understanding we gained from the people we interviewed during our study. They indicate a need for change and identify problem areas that heretofore have not been addressed. We believe that the recommendations are consistent with sound mental-health practices. They reflect the direction toward openness and honesty now associated with sound adoption practice, which we believe is equally applicable to DI.

Some of the new concepts challenge old, ingrained attitudes and practices. They may, indeed, threaten long-held values of society and the institution of marriage and the family as we have known it. Consequently, they may require new and innovative approaches that go beyond many of the ideas and concepts familiar to us today. We leave that to future generations.

In the previous thirteen chapters, we introduced the reader to people who live in the world of donor insemination. Through the stories in Chapters 1 through 11, we sought to bring alive their reactions to the DI experience. After each story, we included a brief commentary with which to highlight some of the important implications. In Chapter 12, we offered our suggestions for sharing the truth of DI with donor offspring and for opening up the subject for all of the people involved. In Chapter 13, we briefly discussed the connection between DI and other high-tech baby-making methods.

Our study, as we have described earlier, was an exploratory project. It was not a scientific or statistical study. The secrecy of the subject denied us such an investigation. Instead, we have perceived our work as a clinical and descriptive foundation upon which we hope that others will be able to build.

For clarity, we have divided our recommendations into four sections: (1) The Donor Offspring, (2) The Parents, (3) The Genetic Donor Father, and (4) The DI Provider of Service.

THE DONOR OFFSPRING

1. Must be accepted as having two genetic parents who are important to him; they contribute to his identity and self-concept. They connect him to his biological and historical past and provide him with information that is vital to his health and well-being.

2. Has a right to know, at an appropriate age, of his DI conception.

3. Has a right to know the identity of the donor father and his medical, social, and familial information.

4. Has a right to meet his donor father if he wishes to have personal contact.

THE PARENTS

1. Must be accepted as the legal, nurturing, and psychological parents of their child. Their role as the rearing parents who protect, provide, and integrate the child into their extended families, both genetic and nongenetic, is of primary importance in the child's development of a self-concept and a standard of values.

2. Must accept the importance of the donor father as the genetic father of their child.

3. Have a right to complete information, including identity, on the donor father, with assurances of lifelong cooperation on his part to be available to the family and the child as needed.

4. Have a responsibility to provide their child with complete information, including the identity of the donor father, and to be supportive in helping the child integrate the knowledge.

5. Have a responsibility to accept and support their child's desire to meet his genetic father at an appropriate age.

THE GENETIC DONOR FATHER

1. Must accept the lifelong responsibility he bears as a genetic parent of a donor offspring. Providing sperm for insemination carries with it the acceptance of the fact that the donor is half of the biological inheritance of the child produced. That acceptance in turn carries with it a solemn obligation to fulfill the responsibilities inherent to being a genetic donor father.

2. Must provide full and complete medical, social, and familial information to the family, and must see that it is updated throughout his lifetime.

3. Must be available to the donor offspring and his family for personal contact if necessary and desired.

4. Has a right to meet the prospective parents of his genetic offspring.

5. Has a right to be told about the outcome of the inseminations and the number of offspring conceived and born of his sperm.

6. Has a right to request current information regarding his genetic offspring.

7. Has a right to request personal contact with his offspring at an appropriate age.

8. Has no financial or legal obligations to the genetic donor offspring.

THE DI PROVIDER OF SERVICE

1. Must accept the concept that the donor is and remains forever half of the child's genetic inheritance. This genetic inheritance is of primary importance because it provides the offspring with medical, historical, and social connections to his origins, and is an integral part of the individual's self-concept. Providing sperm for insemination, therefore, must be viewed as a serious, responsible, carefully administered and documented process, which has lifelong implications for all of the parties involved.

2. Must accept only those sperm donors who are willing to accept responsibility for being known and available genetic fathers to their offspring.

3. Must accept only those sperm donors who voluntarily, without compensation, wish to become genetic fathers.

4. Must employ the highest professional standards of medical and genetic screening of the donor.

5. Must obtain complete medical, social, and familial history of the donor.

6. Must maintain complete records of the donor and the recipients, making such records available to both parties as requested.

7. Must use only one donor's sperm for each insemination. Mixing sperm must be discontinued.

8. Must use only sperm that is known and identified with a specific donor. Anonymous sperm, currently stored, must be destroyed.

9. Must limit the donor to three offspring. This number is lower than the Warnock Commission in England of ten and the American Fertility Society of fifteen. Their recommendations were based on the fear of inbreeding and incest. Our recommendation is related to the concept that

171

each donor should be known and available to his off-spring.

10. Must accept the concept of personal meetings between prospective parents and donors.

11. Must provide the donors and families with identifying information in order to facilitate future contacts.

12. Must recognize that donor insemination is a complex process with lifelong emotional and psychological implications for the participants. Providers must be prepared to facilitate appropriate services such as support groups, individual and family counseling, as well as educational programs for the community.

AFTERWORD

Writers and researchers are frequently guilty of glorifying the importance of their work and its "place in the sun." However, overinvolvement may well be a necessary ingredient in the process of achieving the commitment that leads to successful completion of a project. On a rational level, we have no yardstick by which to measure either the immediate or the long-range value of this book. We have no way of knowing whether or not our recommendations will have an influence on the practices currently in use for donor insemination.

Without a doubt, the growing assessment of high-tech pregnancies and their effect on individuals and on society as a whole indicates a positive and forward-looking focus. At the beginning of this book, we indicated our belief that donor insemination, the oldest method of alternative conception known, provided a good avenue toward an understanding of the complexities and unsolved problems. We deplored the past century's secrecy on the subject and said that we hoped our project could initiate efforts to open up that forbidden world, as well as point to a sounder direction for emerging fertility methodologies.

As this manuscript approached publication, we saw increasing public awareness of the need to consider ethical and moral issues inherent in alternative conceptions and gestations. We read relevant reports in the newspapers almost daily. State legislative committees debate the question of controls on surrogate parenting. Medical societies discuss guidelines for candidates of in-vitro fertilization. Legal groups ponder the dilemma of inherited ownership of frozen fertilized embryos. There is a continuous interest in interviewing the individuals involved.

During the past decade, we have been able to evaluate the importance to readers of a book specifically designed to open up secret areas. In the aftermath of the publication of *The Adoption Triangle*, we heard from thousands of individuals whose lives paralleled those of the people they read about in the book. Many who had lived silently with their solitary feelings experienced the awesome discovery that others had similar feelings. It literally changed their lives, and they came forward to thank us. That new awareness led them, in many instances, to further involvement and openness. They formed groups or joined existing organizations wherein they discussed their status and identity. They lobbied for their rights and for new regulations. They helped others and became experts on the subject. The long-term effect on the professional community was equally profound. Social workers, psychotherapists, administrators, and researchers brought new insights to the field of adoption.

It seems clear to us that *Lethal Secrets* gives many readers the same opportunity that *The Adoption Triangle* offered. If this book can meaningfully touch the life of even one person who heretofore has felt alone with feelings of deprivation and isolation, we will have accomplished a great deal. Further, if reading *Lethal Secrets* prompts members of the donor-insemination family to become open and to share their experiences with others, the book will have succeeded. Still further, if those readers are inspired to play a role in altering the future practices of alternative conception and become active participants in the espousal of change, we will have succeeded far beyond our expectations.

We thank you for being our audience and for hearing us out on a subject we think is of vital importance.

BIBLIOGRAPHY

Alexander, N. J., and Kay, R. (1977). "Antigenicity of Frozen and Fresh Spermatozoa." *Fertility and Sterility*, 28 (11):1234–7.

American Academy of Pediatrics (1983). "How and When to Tell the Adoptee." *News and Comment*, 34:8.

Anglim, E. (1965). "The Adopted Child's Heritage—Two Natural Parents." *Child Welfare*, 44:339–43.

Annas G. J. (1980). "Fathers Anonymous: Beyond the Best Interests of the Sperm Donor." *Fam. Law Q.*, Spring: 14:1–13.

Annas, G., and Elias, S. (Summer 1983). "In Vitro Fertilization and Embryo Transfer: Medicolegal Aspects of a New Technique to Create a Family." *Fam. Law Q.*, XVII: 199–223.

Annas, G. J. (1979). "Artificial Insemination: Beyond the Best Interests of the Donor." *Hastings Center Report*, 9 (4):14–15.

Arditti, R., Klein, R. D., and Minden, S. (1984). *Test-Tube Women: What Future For Motherhood?* London, Eng.: Pandora Press.

Asch, S. S., and Rubin, L. J. (1974). "Postpartum Reactions: Some Unrecognized Variations." *Am. J. of Psych.*: 131:870–74.

Atallah, L. (1976). "Report from a Test-Tube Baby." *NY Times Mag.*, Apr. 18: 16–17, 48–51.

Bache-Wiig, B. (1975). "Adoption Insights: A Course for Adoptive Parents." *Children Today*, 4 (1):22–25.

Baran, A., Pannor, R., and Sorosky, A. D. (1977). "The Lingering Pain of Surrendering a Child." *Psychology Today*, 11 (1):58–60, 88.

———. (1974). "Adoptive Parents and the Sealed Record Controversy."

Social Casework, 55:531–36.

——. (1976). "Open Adoption." *Social Work*, 21:97–100.

Baran, A., Sorosky, A.D., and Pannor, R. (1975). "Secret Adoption Records: the Dilemma of Our Adoptees." *Psychology Today*, 9 (7):38–42, 96–98.

Barinbaum, L. (1974). "Identity Crisis in Adolescence: the Problem of an Adopted Girl." *Adolescence*, 9:547–54.

Barton, M., Walker, K., and Weisner, B. P. (1945). "Artificial Insemination." *Brit. Med. J.*, 1 (1):3–40.

Beck, W. W. (1974). "Artificial Insemination and Semen Preservation." *Clinical Obst. and Gyn.*, 17 (4):115–25.

Beck, William W., Jr. (1976). "A Critical Look at the Legal, Ethical and Technical Aspects of Artificial Insemination." *Fertility and Sterility*, 27, No. 1.

Bell, C. J. (1986). "Adoptive Pregnancy: Legal and Social Work Issues." *Child Welfare*, 65 (5):421–435.

Berger, D. M. (1982). "Psychological Implications of Donor Insemination." *Int. J. Psych. Med.*, 12:49–77.

Berman, S. J. (1979). "Artificial Insemination and Public Policy." *NE J. of Med.*, 300, No. 11.

Black, J. A., and Stone, F. H. (1958). "Medical Aspects of Adoption." *Lancet*, 2:1272–75.

Black, R. (Nov.–Dec. 1984). "Critique: A Genetic Counseling Casebook." *Social Work* 29: 565.

Blacker, C. P. (1957). "Artificial Insemination (Donor)." *Eugenics Rev.*, 48 (4):209–11.

Bodenheimer, B. M. (1975). "New Trends and Requirements in Adoption Law and Proposals for Legislative Change." *S. Cal. Law Rev.*, 49:10–109.

Bok, S. (1978). "Lying to Children: The Risks of Paternalism." *Hastings Center Rep.*, 8 (3):10–13.

Borgatta, E.F., and Fanshel, D. (1965). *Behavioral Characteristics of Children Known to Psychiatric Out-Patient Clinics.* New York: Child Welfare League of America.

Breasted, M. (1977). "Babybrokers Reaping Huge Fees." *New York Times*, June 28:1, 11.

Brown, J. L. (1974). "Rootedness." *Involvement: The Family Resource Magazine*, May–June:1–7.

Burke, C. (1975). "The Adult Adoptee's Constitutional Right to Know His Origins." *S. Cal. Law Rev.*, 48:1196–1220.

Cadoret, R. J., Cunningham, L., Loftus, R., and Edwards, J. E. (1975). "Studies of Adoptees from Psychiatrically Disturbed Biological Parents, II: Temperamental, Hyperactive, Antisocial and Developmental Variables." *J. of Pediatrics*, 87:301–6.

Cary, W. (1948). "Results of Artificial Insemination With an Extra-marital Specimen (Semi-Adoption)." *Am. J. of Obst. and Gyn.* 56 (3):727–32.

Clamar, A. (1980). "Psychological Implications of Donor Insemination." *Am. J. Psychoanal.,* 40:173–7.

Clamar, A. (1984). "Artificial Insemination by Donor: the Anonymous Pregnancy." *Am. J. Forens. Psychol.,* 2:27–37.

Crowe, R. R. (1974). "An Adoption Study of Antisocial Personality." *Arch. of Gen. Psychiatry,* 31:785–91.

Curie-Cohen, M., Luttrell, M., and Shapiro, S. (1979). "Current Practice of Artificial Insemination by Donor in the United States." *NE J. of Med.* 300:585–620.

David, A., and Avidan, D. (1976). "Artificial Insemination Donor: Clinical and Psychological Aspects." *Fertil. Steril.,* 27:528.

Davis, J. H. (1979). "The Pediatric Role in Adoption." *Clin. Pediatr.,* 7:439–43.

Dawkins, S. (1972). "The Pre-Adopter and Infertility." *Child Adoption,* 67:24–32.

Dienes, A. (1968). "Artificial Donor Insemination: Perspectives on Legal and Social Change." *Iowa Law Rev.,* 54, 253–269.

Dixon, R. E., and Buttram, V. C. (1976). "Artificial Insemination Using Donor Semen: a Review of 171 Cases." *Fertility and Sterility,* 27 (2):130–4.

Dunstan, G. R. (1975). "Ethical Aspects of Donor Insemination." *J. of Med. Ethics,* 1, 1, 42–44.

Dusky, L. (1975). "The Adopted Child Has a Right to Know Everything." *Parents' Mag.,* Oct.:40–43, 64.

Eiduson, B. T., and Livermore, J.B. (1952). "Complications in Therapy With Adopted Children." *Am. J. of Orthopsych.,* 23:795–802.

Elias, E., and Annas, G. J. (1986). "Social Policy Considerations in Noncoital Reproduction." *JAMA,* 255:62–8.

Elonen, A. S., and Schwartz, E. M. (1969). "A Longitudinal Study of the Emotional, Social and Academic Functioning of Adopted Children." *Child Welfare,* 48:72–78.

Erikson, E. H. (1968). *Identity: Youth and Crisis.* New York: W. W. Norton.

Farris, E., and Garrison, M. (1954). "Emotional Impact of Successful Donor Insemination." *Obst. and Gyn.,* 3 (1):19–20.

Finegold, W. J. (1964). *Artificial Insemination.* Springfield, Ill.: Charles C. Thomas.

Fisher, F. (1973). *The Search for Anna Fisher.* New York: Arthur Fields.

Fletcher, J. (1974). *The Ethics of Genetic Control.* Garden City, N.Y.: Anchor Books/Anchor Press, p. 40.

Freedman, J. (1977). "Notes For Practice: an Adoptee in Search of Identity." *Social Work,* 22:227–29.

BIBLIOGRAPHY

Freeman, J. T. (1970). "Who Am I? Where Did I Come From? Girl's Search for Real Mother." *Ladies' Home J.*, Mar.:74, 132–36.

Freud, S. (1909). "Family Romances." Reprinted in J. Strachey, ed., *Collected Papers*, Vol. 5. London: Hogarth Press, 1950. Pp. 74–78.

Frey, K. (Winter 1982). "New Reproductive Technologies: The Legal Problem and a Solution." *Tenn. Law Rev.* 49:303–342.

Frisk, M. (1964). "Identity Problems and Confused Conceptions of the Genetic Ego in Adopted Children During Adolescence." *Acta Paedo Psychiatrica*, 31:6–12.

Gawronski, A., Landgreen, L., and Schneider, C. (1974). "Adoptees' Curiosity about Origins—a Search for Identity." Unpublished master's thesis, Univ. of So. Cal. Sch. of Soc. Work.

Gaylord, C. L. (1976). "The Adoptive Child's Right to Know." *Case and Comment*, Mar.–Apr.:38–44.

Gerstel, G. (1963). "A Psychoanalytic View of Artificial Donor Insemination." *Am. J. of Psychotherapy*, 17:64–77.

Glatzer, H. T. (1955). "Adoption and Delinquency." *Nervous Child*, 11:52–56.

Goldstein, J., Freud, A., and Solnit, A. J. (1973). *Beyond the Best Interests of the Child*. New York: Free Press.

Guttmacher, A. F. (1960). "The Role of Artificial Insemination in the Treatment of Sterility." *Obst. and Gyn. Survey*, 15:767–85.

Haley, A. (1976). *Roots*. New York: Doubleday.

Handy, E. S. C., and Pukui, M. K. (1958). "The Polynesian Family System in Ka-'U, Hawaii." Wellington, NZ.: *Polynesian Soc.* Pp. 71, 72.

Hanson, F. H., and Rock, J. (1950). "Effect of Adoption on Fertility and Other Reproductive Functions." *Am. J. of Obst. and Gyn.*, 59:311–20.

Hill, A. M. (1970). "Experiences with Artificial Insemination." *Australia and NZ. J. of Obst. and Gyn.*, 10:112–14.

Howard, M. (1975). "I Take After Somebody; I Have Real Relatives; I Possess a Real Name." *Psychology Today*, 12:33, 35–37.

Kiester, E. (1974). "Should We Unlock the Adoption files?" *Today's Health*, 8:54–60.

Kleegman, S., Amelar, R. D., Sherman, J. K., Hirshhorn, K., and Pilpel, H. (1970). "Artificial Donor Insemination: Round Table." *Med. Aspects of Human Sexuality*, 5:85–111.

Klibanoff, E. B. (1977). "Roots: An Adoptee's Quest." *Harvard Law Sch. Bulletin*, 28, No. 3:34–40.

Kornitzer, M. (1971). "The Adopted Adolescent and the Sense of Identity." *Child Adoption*, 66:43–48.

Kovacs, G.T., Clayton, C. E., and McGowan, P. (1983). "The Attitudes of Semen Donors." *Clin. Reprod. Fertility*, 2:73–5.

Kraus, J., and Quinn, P. E. (1977). "Human Artificial Insemination—Some Social and Legal Issues." *Med. J. Aust.*, 1:710.

BIBLIOGRAPHY

Kremer J., Frijling, B. W., and Nass, J. L. (1984). "Psychosocial Aspects of Parenthood by Artificial Insemination by Donor." *Lancet,* 83:628.

Lamson, H. D., Pinard, W. J., and Meaker, S. E. (1951). "Sociologic and Psychologic Aspects of Artificial Insemination With Donor Semen." *JAMA,* 145:1062–4.

Ledward, R. S., Symonds, E. M., and Eynon, S. (1982). "Social and Environmental Factors as Criteria for Success in Artificial Insemination by Donor (AID)." *J. Biosoc. Sci.,* 14:263–75.

LeShan, E. J. (1977). "Should Adoptees Search for Their 'Real' Parents?" *Woman's Day,* 3:8:40, 214, 218.

Lewis, H. N. (1971). "The Psychiatric Aspects of Adoption." In J. G. Howells, ed., *Modern Perspectives in Child Psychiatry.* New York: Brunner/Mazel. Pp. 428–51.

Lifshitz, M., Baum, R., Balgur, I., and Cohen, C. (1975). "The Impact of the Social Milieu Upon the Nature of Adoptee's Emotional Difficulty." *J. of Marriage and the Fam.,* 2:221–28.

Lifton, B. J. (1975). *Twice Born: Memoirs of an Adopted Daughter.* New York: McGraw-Hill.

Lifton, B. J. (1977). "My Search for My Roots." *Seventeen,* 3:132, 133, 164, 165.

Lifton, R. J. (1974). Testimony, "In the Matter of Ann Carol S." Atty, Gertrud Mainzer. Surrogate's Ct., Bronx Cty., NY.

Lifton, R.J. (1976). "On the Adoption Experience." Foreword to M. K. Benet, *The Politics of Adoption.* New York: Free Press. Pp. 1–7.

Lion, A. (1976). "A Survey of Fifty Adult Adoptees Who Used the Rights of the Israel 'Open File' Adoption Law." Paper presented at the annual meeting of the International Forum on Adolescence, Jerusalem, Israel.

Mazor, M. D. (May 1979). "Barren Couples." *Psychology Today,* pp. 101–112.

McKuen, R. (1976). *Finding My Father: One Man's Search for Identity.* Los Angeles: Cheval Books/Coward, McCann & Geoghegan.

Menning, B. E. (1975). "The Infertile Couple: a Plea for Advocacy." *Child Welfare,* 54:454-60.

Milsom, I., and Bergman, P. (1982). "A study of Parental Attitudes After Donor Insemination (AID)." *Acta Obstet. Gynecol. Scan.,* 61:125–8.

O'Rourke, S. M. (1985). "Family Law in a Brave New World: Private Ordering of Parental Rights and Responsibilities for Donor Insemination." *Berkeley Women's Law J.,* 1:140–174.

Pannor, R., and Baran, A. (May–June 1984). "Open Adoption as Standard Practice." *Child Welfare* 63 (10):245–247.

Pannor, R., and Nerlove, E. A. (1987). "Group Therapy with Adopted Adolescents and Their Parents." Paper presented at the annual meeting of the Institute for Clinical Social Work, San Francisco, Calif.

Pannor, R., Baran, A., and Sorosky, A. D. (1976a). "Attitudes of Birth Parents, Adoptive Parents and Adoptees Toward the Sealed Adoption

Record." *J. of the Ontario Assoc. of Children's Aid Societies*, 19, No. 4:1–7.

Pannor, R., Massarik, F., and Evans, B. W. (1971). *The Unmarried Father*. New York: Springer.

Pannor, R., Sorosky, A. D., and Baran, A. (1974). "Opening the Sealed Record in Adoption: the Human Need for Continuity." *J. of Jewish Communal Service*, 51:188–96.

Parker, P. J. (1982). "Surrogate Motherhood: the Interaction of Litigation, Legislation and Psychiatry." *Int. J. Law Psyc.*, 5:341–54.

Paton, J. M. (1954). *The Adopted Break Silence*. Acton, Calif.: Life History Study Center.

Pies, C. (1985). *Considering Parent Hood: A Workbook for Lesbians*. San Francisco: Spinsters Ink.

Prager, B., and Rothstein, S. A. (1973). "The Adoptee's Right to Know His Natural Heritage." *New York Law Forum*, 19:137–56.

Quindlen, A. (1987). "The Try-Everything World of Baby Craving." *Life Magazine*, June: 30–34.

Reading, A.E., Sledmere, C. M., and Cox, D.N. (1982). "A Survey of Patient Attitudes Toward Artificial Insemination by Donor." *J. Psychosomatic Res.*, 26:429–33.

Reynolds, W. F., and Chiappise, D. (1975). "The Search by Adopted Persons for Their Natural Parents: a Research Project Comparing Those Who Search and Those Who Do Not." Paper presented at meeting of Am. Psychology-Law Soc., Chicago, Ill.

Richardson, J. W. (1987). "The Role of a Psychiatric Consultation To an Artifical Insemination by Donor Program." *Psychiatric Annals*, 17:2, Feb.

Robinson, S., and Pizer, H. F. (1985). *Having a Baby Without a Man*. New York: Simon and Schuster.

Rowland, R., and Ruffin, C. (1983). "Community Attitudes to Artificial Insemination by Husband or Donor, In Vitro Fertilization, and Adoption." *Clin. Reprod. Fertil.* 2:195–206.

Rubin, B. (1965). "Psychological Aspects of Human Artifical Insemination." *Arch. of Gen. Psychiatry*, 13:121–32.

Sants, H. J. (1965). "Genealogical Bewilderment in Children With Substitute Parents." *Child Adoption*, 47:32–42.

Schechter, M. D. (1960). "Observations on Adopted Children." *Arch. of Gen. Psychiatry*, 3:21–32.

Simmons, F. A. (1957). "The Role of the Husband in Therapeutic Donor Insemination." *Fertility and Sterility*, 8 (6):547–50.

Smith, G. P. (1980). "Great Expectations of Convoluted Realities: Artificial Insemination Influx." *Family Law Rev.*, 3:37–44.

Snowden, R., and Mitchell, G. D. (1983). *The Artificial Family: A Consideration of Artificial Insemination by Donor*. London, Eng.: Counterpoint.

181

BIBLIOGRAPHY

Sokoloff, M. Z. (1987). "Alternative Methods of Reproduction: Effects on the Child." *Clinical Pediatrics*, 26 (1):11–17.

Sorosky, A. D., Baran, A., and Pannor, R. (1974). "The Reunion of Adoptees and Birth Relatives." *J. of Youth and Adolesc.*, 3:195–206.

———. (1975). "Identity Conflicts in Adoptees." *Am. J. of Orthopsychiatry*, 45:18–27.

———. (1976). "The Effects of the Sealed Record in Adoption." *Am. J. of Psych.*, 133:900–4.

———. (1977). "Adoption and the Adolescent: An Overview." In S. C. Feinstein and P. Giovacchini, eds., *Adolescent Psychiatry*, 5. New York: Jason Aronson. Pp. 54–72.

———. (1978). "Adopted Children." In D. Cantwell and P. Tanguagy, eds., *Clinical Child Psych..* Jamaica, NY.: Spectrum Publications, forthcoming.

———. (1981). "Infertility, Adoption, and Artificial Insemination." In Pasnau R., ed., *Psychosocial Aspects of Medical Practices.* Menlo Park: Addison-Wesley Press. Pp. 16–26.

———. (1984 2nd Ed.). *The Adoption Triangle: Sealed or Open Records: How They Affect Adoptees, Birth Parents, and Adoptive Parents.* New York: Anchor Press-Doubleday.

Sorosky, A. D., et al. (1977). "Adoption and the Adolescent: An Overview." *Adolescent Psychiatry*, 5. New York: Jason Aronson. Pp. 54–72.

———. (1975). "The Psychological Effects of the Sealed Record on Adoptive Parents." *World J. of Psychosynthesis*, 7 (6):13–18.

Stewart C., Daniels, K., and Boulnois, J. D. (1982). "The Development of a Psychosocial Approach to Artificial Insemination of Donor Sperm." *NZ Med. J.*, 95:853–6.

Teresi, D., and McAuliffe, K. (1985). "Male Pregnancy." *Omni Mag.*, 8(3):91–97.

Triseliotis, J. (1973). *In Search of Origins: The Experiences of Adopted People.* London: Routledge and Kegan Paul.

Tyler, E. T. (1973). "The Clinical Use of Frozen Semen Banks." *Fertility and Sterility*, 24 (5):413–16.

Wallis, C. (Sept. 1984). "Making Babies: The New Science of Conception." *Time Mag.*, 124:46–56.

Walters, W. W., and Sousa-Posa, J. (1966). "Psychiatric Aspects of Artificial Insemination (Donor)." *J. Can. Med. Assoc.*, 95:106.

Waltzer, H. (1982). "Psychological and Legal Aspects of Artificial Insemination (AID): An Overview." *Am. J. Psychother.*, 36(1):91–102.

Weinstein, E. A. (1962). "Adoption and Infertility." *Am. Sociological Rev.*, 27:408–12.

Wellisch, E. (1952). "Children Without Genealogy: A Problem of Adoption." *Mental Health*, 13:41–42.

Wessel, M. A. (1960). "The Pediatrician and Adoption." *NE J. of Med.*, 262:446–50.

BIBLIOGRAPHY

Wieder, H. (1977a). "On Being Told of Adoption." *The Psychoanalytic Q.*, 46:1–22.

Wieder, H. (1977b). "The Family Romance Fantasies of Adopted Children." *Psychoanalytic Q.*, 46:185–200.

Winslade, W. J. (1981). "Surrogate Mothers: Private Right or Public Wrong?" *J. Med. Ethics*, 7:143–4.

INDEX

INDEX

Donor offspring
  on being told, 68–70
  divorce and, 71–72
  feelings of, 59, 60, 62–63, 64
  on finding real fathers, 66–68, 72–73
  interview with, 55–70
  on learning the truth, 57–58, 60, 62, 63–64, 66, 83
  openness/honesty, importance of, 155
  reasons for being told, 71
  search for truth, case example, 74–83
  secrecy, effects of, 52, 68–70
  telling about conception, suggestions for, 155–161
Donors
  characteristics of, 90
  doctors as, 97
  emotional aspects, case example, 89–96
  meeting children, 106
  pre-donation testing, 91–92
  pros/cons of donating sperm, 90
  screening of, 29
  women's fantasies about, 29–30, 33

F

Fathers of donor offspring
  ambivalent feelings of, 43–45, 71
  distance from children, 45–47
  role in family, 51, 77, 84
Frozen sperm, 119
Future technology, 162–166
  baby making as big business, 164–165
  male pregnancy, 163

G

Gay men, as donors, 127, 137
Genetic disorders, and insemination decision, 60–63, 99–108

I

Incest, in donor insemination families, 65–66, 72
Infertility
  blaming woman for, 24–25
  male-female percentage of, 25
  See also Male infertility.
Infidelity, equated with DI, 37–38

L

Lesbian couples
  attitude about negative reactions, 134–135
  birth certificate issue, 134
  case examples, 122–130
  donor, relationship to, 136–137
  donors and AIDS, 137
  emotional stability of children raised by, 130–131
  gay men, as donors, 127, 137
  and identity of donor, 132–134, 137
  telling child about conception, 160–161

M

Male infertility
  environmental causes, 25
  man's feelings about, 25, 31
  mourning process and, 36, 37, 52
  secrecy about, 23–24, 26, 27–28
  woman's feelings about, 25–26
Mothers of donor offspring, as "real" parent, 45–46, 51, 84
Mourning, and infertility, 36, 37, 52

P

Power, parental, DI families, 51, 77, 84
Pregnancy, man's feelings during, 34–35, 38–39

186